The Unseen March

The Unseen March

Wayne A Ince

Prologue

My Rucksack

The desert sand of Kuwait, 1991, wasn't just sand. It was a fine, talcum-powder grit that got into everything—my weapon, my teeth, the creases of the letters from home. For me, it was the taste of Desert Storm, a chaotic roar of liberation and fear, my first direct experience in the concussive symphony of war. I returned from deployment, changed but functional, told to carry on. My rucksack, a backpack, grew heavier with each deployment. In Bosnia (1995-96), the weight was the eerie silence of mass graves and the hollow eyes of children in a fractured land. In Kosovo (1999), it was the tension of peacekeeping in a war zone, the constant threat of asymmetric conflict, and the moral ambiguity of intervention. For Operation Uphold Democracy in Haiti (1994), the burdens were the oppressive heat, the palpable instability, and the strain of being both protector and occupier in a jungle landscape.

Each mission added a stone to my rucksack: fear, grief, hyper-vigilance, a deep-seated unease. The military taught me to pack my gear efficiently, but no one taught me how to unpack my mind.

After 23 years of honorable service, culminating in my retirement as a Senior Master Sergeant, I, Wayne, affectionately known as "Big Sarge," swapped my military uniform for civilian attire. However, the backpack was still there, though unseen. The world witnessed a competent and self-controlled individual who withstood work stress carrying an invisible load on my shoulders – my rucksack.

Inside, a car backfiring was an ambush. A crowded mall required a tactical scan of exits and threats. I don't like malls. Emotional numbness created a chasm between the family I loved more than anything and me. The very skills that kept my brothers and me alive overseas—hyper-awareness, emotional control, readiness for threat—were strangling my life at home. The delayed onset of my

Post-Traumatic Stress Disorder wasn't a failure; it was my mind and body, finally in a perceived safe zone, beginning the long-overdue process of dealing with the accumulated trauma of a career in service.

This book exists because of my journey and the journeys of thousands like me- not just veterans, but the law enforcement officers who have seen too much violence, the firefighter who carries the memories of lives they couldn't save, and the family members whose home fronts become secondary theaters of a silent war.

This is not a book about erasing my past. It is a manual for managing the weight of my rucksack, for learning how to unpack it piece by piece, with intention and support, so I can finally stand tall without being pulled down by the unseen load. The march continues, but it doesn't have to be a forced march through hell. It can become a walk toward peace. I have faith and believe in my journey to wellness.

Gear up. The march continues.

A Note to the Reader

Welcome. If you're holding this book, you or someone you care about is likely carrying a heavy load. This guide is designed to be a tool, not a cure. It is divided into parts that you can approach in order, or you can jump to the sections that speak to your most immediate needs—especially Part IV: Crisis Management.

The language is direct, avoiding unnecessary clinical jargon. You'll find exercises, strategies, and resources drawn from evidence-based practices and the hard-won wisdom of those who've walked this path.

Most importantly, this book comes from a place of deep respect. Your experiences are valid. Your reactions are understandable adaptations to extraordinary stress. Our goal is not to judge those adaptations, but to help you build new ones that serve you better in the life you have now.

You are not broken. You are adapting. Let's adapt together. Don't have to us AI for answers. I didn't.

A note on the language of this book: you will find tactical framing throughout—words like "mission," "terrain," and "fortify." This is intentional. Familiar language can make unfamiliar territory more navigable. But understand this clearly: the mission we are engaged in together is not one of brute force or toughing it out. It is a mission of self-compassion and vulnerability—the kind of courage that takes more genuine strength than any firefight. You are not being asked to fight harder. You are being asked to feel, to reach out, and to heal.

How to Use This Book

Go At Your Own Pace. This is not a race. Some chapters may take a day, others a week. Honor your process.

Use the Worksheets and examples. Writing is a powerful tool for processing and tracking progress. There is also an accompanying app you may use.

Jump to Crisis Help First. If you are in acute distress, go directly to Chapter 15 and Chapter 17 for immediate resources and agency contacts.

Involve Your Support System. Consider sharing relevant chapters (like Chapter 10 on relationships) with a trusted partner or family member.

This is a Supplement, Not a Replacement. This book is designed to complement professional therapy and medical care, not replace it. Always seek professional medical advice especially when in distress.

PART I

Understanding the Terrain

Before you can begin to heal, you need to understand what you're carrying. Part I lays the groundwork: what PTSD actually is at the neurological level, how it arrives through the many different roads of service, and why the hardest first step—accepting the weight without surrendering to it—is also the most essential. You cannot unpack a rucksack you have never opened. These chapters open it.

1

Chapter 1: What is PTSD? Beyond the Diagnosis

You've likely heard the term: Post-Traumatic Stress Disorder. It's a clinical diagnosis from the DSM-5, the manual mental health professionals use. But for those living with it, PTSD is less a "disorder" and more an injury—an injury to your stress response system, your memory processing, and your sense of safety.

The Neurobiology of Survival

When you experience extreme trauma, your brain's alarm system—the amygdala—goes into overdrive. It shouts "THREAT!" to the rest of your body, flooding you with stress hormones like cortisol and adrenaline. This is the brilliant, ancient fight-flight-freeze-fawn response that saves lives in acute danger.

In PTSD, this alarm system becomes faulty. It gets stuck in the "on" position or fires at the slightest provocation. A slamming door, a specific smell, a tone of voice, a date on the calendar—these become tripwires that trigger the full survival response, even though you are physically safe. Meanwhile, the hippocampus (which helps file mem-

6

ories as "past events") and the prefrontal cortex (which handles rational thought and moderation) can become impaired, making it hard to convince your nervous system that the danger is over.

The Symptom Clusters (In Plain Language)

The DSM-5 groups PTSD symptoms into four clusters:

Interference: Yesterday's events impact today. This includes flashbacks (feeling like you're reliving it), nightmares, and intrusive, distressing memories.

Avoidance: Steering clear of anything that might trigger those intrusions. This means avoiding people, places, conversations, thoughts, or feelings associated with the trauma. It's a logical but isolating strategy.

Negative Alterations in Cognitions and Mood: This is the shadow cast on your worldview. It can include:

Inability to recall key features of the trauma.

Persistent negative beliefs about yourself, others, or the world ("I am broken," "The world is utterly dangerous," "No one can be trusted").

Distorted blame of self or others.

Persistent negative emotions (fear, horror, anger, guilt, shame).

Loss of interest in activities you once enjoyed.

Feeling detached or estranged from others.

Alterations in Arousal and Reactivity: Your body stays on high alert.

This includes:

Irritability and angry outbursts.

Reckless or self-destructive behavior.

Hypervigilance (constantly scanning for danger).

Exaggerated startle response.

Problems with concentration.

Sleep disturbance.

Why Understanding This Matters

Knowing this isn't about labeling yourself. It's about demystifying your experience. That panic attack in the grocery store isn't a character flaw; it's a triggered survival response. The anger that flares is often fear in body armor. The numbness is a protective circuit breaker. When you see your reactions as symptoms of an injury rather than personal failings, you can begin to address them with clarity and self-compassion, not shame.

WAYNE'S INSIGHT

"For years, I just thought I was an angry guy with a bad memory who couldn't sleep. When a therapist explained it as my body being stuck in a combat zone, even in my living room, it was the first time I didn't feel crazy. I felt injured. And injuries can be treated."

Chapter 1 End Notes & References

LeDoux, J. E. (2000). Emotion circuits in the brain. Annual Review of Neuroscience.

Bremner, J. D. (2006). Traumatic stress: effects on the brain. Dialogues in Clinical Neuroscience.

American Psychiatric Association. (2022). Diagnostic and Statistical

Manual of Mental Disorders, Fifth Edition, Text Revision (DSM-5-TR).

Van der Kolk, B. A. (2014). The Body Keeps the Score: Brain, Mind, and Body in the Healing of Trauma. Viking.

U.S. Department of Veterans Affairs. (2023). PTSD: National Center for PTSD. https://www.ptsd.va.gov/

2

Chapter 2: The Many Faces of Service

While the core symptoms of PTSD are universal, the paths that lead to it are shaped by your role and experiences. Understanding your specific "pathway" can help tailor your recovery.

The Military Veteran's Path

Combat Trauma: Direct engagement, witnessing death/injury, fearing for one's life, causing harm. This includes the moral injury of actions taken or not taken in war.

Operational Stress: The cumulative grind of deployments: constant vigilance, harsh conditions, separation, and the paradox of being both powerful and powerless.

Military Sexual Trauma (MST): A profound betrayal within the unit structure. MST stands apart from other forms of military trauma in a way that demands specific acknowledgment. When sexual assault or harassment occurs in uniform, the perpetrator is often a fellow service member or superior—someone the survivor was trained to trust with their life. The institution itself, which demands loyalty and offers belonging in return, may have failed to protect or even actively discouraged reporting. This dual betrayal—by a comrade and by the chain of command—can shatter the foundational trust that military culture depends on. It often produces a uniquely complex form of PTSD layered with shame, isolation, and the particular pain of having been harmed inside the family you served. MST survivors deserve to know: your reaction is not weakness. It is a proportionate response to a profound violation of trust.

Loss: The grief of losing comrades, often in violent or sudden ways.

Transition Stress: The identity crisis of leaving the structured, mission-driven world for the ambiguities of civilian life.

The Law Enforcement Officer's Path

Cumulative Exposure: Repeated exposure to violence, tragedy, cruelty, and human suffering. The "routine" call that turns horrific.

Critical Incidents: Officer-involved shootings, severe assaults, high-risk tactical operations, gruesome death scenes.

Organizational Stress: Shift work, bureaucracy, public scrutiny, internal politics, and the "warrior vs. guardian" cultural conflict.

Hyper-Vigilance as a Job Requirement: The necessary skill of threat assessment becomes a hard-to-switch-off default setting, bleeding into home life.

The Fire/Rescue/EMS Path

Traumatic Exposure: Repeatedly attending to severe injuries, death (especially of children), failed rescues, and catastrophic scenes.

Physical Risk & Close Calls: The inherent danger of the job, near-misses, and line-of-duty deaths of colleagues.

Cumulative Grief: Bearing witness to families at their most devastated moments, over and over.

Physiological Stress: Sleep disruption, extreme physical exertion, and exposure to toxins.

The Family Trauma Path (Spouses, Children, Parents)

Secondary Traumatic Stress: Absorbing the emotional residue of a loved one's trauma through their stories, moods, and behaviors.

Direct Trauma: Experiencing the volatility of a loved one's PTSD—outbursts, emotional withdrawal, recklessness—which can itself be traumatic.

Chronic Stress & Role Changes: Living in a constant state of "walking on eggshells," becoming a caregiver, losing emotional and financial stability.

Grief for the "Before": Mourning the person or family life that existed before the trauma.

Common Thread

Across all paths runs the thread of betrayal (by others, by institutions, by one's own body or mind), loss (of safety, of identity, of brethren, of innocence), and the burden of witnessing things that cannot be unseen. Your trauma is valid, regardless of whether it fits a stereotypical image of PTSD. The firefighter haunted by a pediatric code, the veteran with MST, the spouse living in fear of a loved one's night terrors—all are carrying legitimate, heavy stones in their rucksack.

Wayne's Insight

"I am a military veteran. An ordinary citizen with an extraordinary journey. Your path won't be like many others. Also, the time it takes to heal and recover varies from person to person. Your struggle belongs to you just as the victory is unique to you. So please go. Don't let your rucksack weigh you down to the point you stop moving forward. Keep going."

Chapter 2 End Notes & References

Figley, C. R. (Ed.). (1995). Compassion Fatigue: Coping with Secondary Traumatic Stress Disorder in Those Who Treat the Traumatized. Brunner/Mazel.

Litz, B. T., et al. (2009). Moral injury and moral repair in war veterans: A preliminary model and intervention strategy. Clinical Psychology Review.

Violanti, J. M. (2014). Dying for the Job: Police Work Exposure and Health. Charles C Thomas Publisher.

National Fallen Firefighters Foundation. (2022). Trauma and the Firefighter.

3

Chapter 3: The Invisible Wound

If you've made it this far into the book, you've already taken a significant step. You're seeking information, looking for a way forward. But before we get into tools and techniques, we need to address the single biggest barrier to healing: stigma.

The Culture of "Toughness"

Military, law enforcement, and emergency services cultures share a core value: resilience through toughness. You're trained to compartmentalize, to mission-focus through chaos, to be the calm in the storm for others. These are vital, life-saving skills. But they come with a dangerous shadow belief: that acknowledging psychological pain is weakness.

This creates a stark conflict. Seeking help for PTSD, which is difficult for those most at risk, is often avoided because it's perceived as an act of failure. "I've survived firefights, but I can't handle my brain?" "I'm supposed to protect others, and I can't even protect myself from my own memories?"

The Truth About Strength

Here's what needs to be said plainly: Seeking help is not weakness. It is tactical intelligence.

Would you avoid a medic for your leg wound, believing "real warriors don't need doctors"? If your weapon jammed in combat, would you refuse to clear it because "a real soldier would make it work"? Of course not. You'd address the problem with the appropriate tools

PTSD is an injury to your nervous system and your brain's stress-processing capacity. It requires appropriate intervention, just like any other injury. That you should "just get over it" is as absurd—and as dangerous—as telling someone with a compound fracture to "walk it off."

Self-Judgment: The Internal Enemy

External stigma is damaging, but often the harshest critic is the one in your own head. Common self-judgments include:

"I should be over this by now." Trauma doesn't have an expiration date. Healing isn't linear.

"Others had it worse." Trauma is not a competition. Your pain is valid regardless of what someone else endured.

"I'm broken." You are injured, not broken. Injuries heal. Systems adapt.

"If I admit I have PTSD, I'm admitting I failed." PTSD is a byproduct of survival, not failure. It means your nervous system did its job—it kept you alive.

These judgments are rooted in misunderstanding PTSD. They treat it as a moral or character issue when it is a physiological and psychological response to intolerable stress.

Acceptance: The First Mission Objective

Acceptance doesn't mean resignation or defeat. It means acknowledging reality so you can respond effectively.

Acceptance means:

Naming the injury: "I have PTSD" or "I am dealing with trauma responses."

Understanding the cause: "My nervous system was repeatedly exposed to life-threatening or morally injurious events, and it adapted to survive."

Recognizing the symptoms: "These nightmares, this anger, this numbness—these are symptoms, not my identity."

Committing to treatment: "I will use the tools and resources available to me."

Acceptance is not passive. It's the tactical assessment that precedes mission planning. You can't navigate terrain you refuse to acknowledge.

Breaking the Silence

One of the most powerful acts against stigma is simply talking about it.

This doesn't mean you have to broadcast your diagnosis to the world. It means finding one safe person—a trusted friend, a counselor, a peer in a veteran or first responder support group—and saying the words out loud.

"I'm struggling."

"I think I have PTSD."

"I need help."

These sentences, spoken aloud, break isolation. They transform a private shame into a shared burden. And shared burdens are lighter.

Wayne's Insight

"The hardest words I ever said weren't in military service or combat. They were sitting across from my loved one, telling her I wasn't okay and speaking to a psychologist. I'd led combat comm teams through war zones, but I

couldn't lead myself out of my head. Saying it out loud fixed nothing instantly, but it stopped me from carrying it alone. That was the beginning."

Chapter 3 End Notes & References

Bryan, C. J., & Morrow, C. E. (2011). Circumventing mental health stigma by embracing the warrior culture: Lessons learned from the Defender's

Edge program. Professional Psychology: Research and Practice.

Britt, T. W. (2000). The stigma of psychological problems in a work environment: Evidence from the screening of service members returning from Bosnia. Journal of Applied Social Psychology.

Hoge, C. W., et al. (2004). Combat duty in Iraq and Afghanistan, mental health problems, and barriers to care. New England Journal of Medicine.

PART II

Fortifying Your Position—Foundational Skills

Now that we've mapped the terrain of PTSD—what it is, where it comes from, and why your mind and body respond the way they do—the next phase of this mission is to fortify your position. Think of the chapters ahead as field training for your nervous system: the grounding techniques, sleep strategies, and mind-body tools that will stabilize you before deeper work begins. These are not lesser skills. They are the foundation everything else is built on, and they belong in your rucksack long before you move into advanced terrain.

4

Chapter 4: Grounding Techniques

When you're in the grip of a flashback, a panic attack, or severe anxiety, your brain is no longer in the present. It's re-experiencing the past as if it's happening right now. Your sympathetic nervous system has hit the gas pedal, and rational thought has left the building.

Grounding techniques are your immediate, tactical response. They are simple, portable tools that work by re-engaging your senses with the present environment, essentially telling your brain: "You are here. You are safe. The threat is not current."

The 5-4-3-2-1 Sensory Grounding Method

This is the gold standard of grounding techniques because it engages all five senses sequentially, forcing your brain to process current, real-time input.

How to do it:

Five things you can SEE: Look around. Name five objects. Out loud if possible. "I see a blue pen. I see a white wall. I see a brown chair. I see sunlight through the window. I see my watch."

Four things you can TOUCH/FEEL: Physical contact. "I feel my feet on the floor. I feel the chair against my back. I feel my hand on my knee.

I feel the fabric of my jeans."

Three things you can HEAR: Listen actively. "I hear the hum of the air conditioner. I hear traffic outside. I hear my own breathing."

Two things you can SMELL: This one can be harder. "I smell coffee. I smell the faint scent of laundry detergent." If you can't identify two, that's okay—focus on what you can detect.

One thing you can TASTE: Even if it's just the taste in your mouth. "I taste mint from my toothpaste," or "I taste coffee."

Why it works: By engaging your senses deliberately and methodically, you're pulling your brain's processing power out of the trauma memory and into the physical present. You are re-establishing the fact that you are here, not there.

Box Breathing (Tactical Breathing)

This technique is used by military special operations forces to manage acute stress in high-stakes situations. It works by activating the parasympathetic nervous system—the body's "rest and digest" mode—countering the fight-or-flight response.

How to do it:

Inhale through your nose for a count of 4. Slowly. Fill your lungs.

Hold your breath for a count of 4. Not straining, just pausing.

Exhale through your mouth for a count of 4. Slow, controlled release.

Hold empty for a count of 4. Before the next inhale.

Repeat for 3-5 cycles.

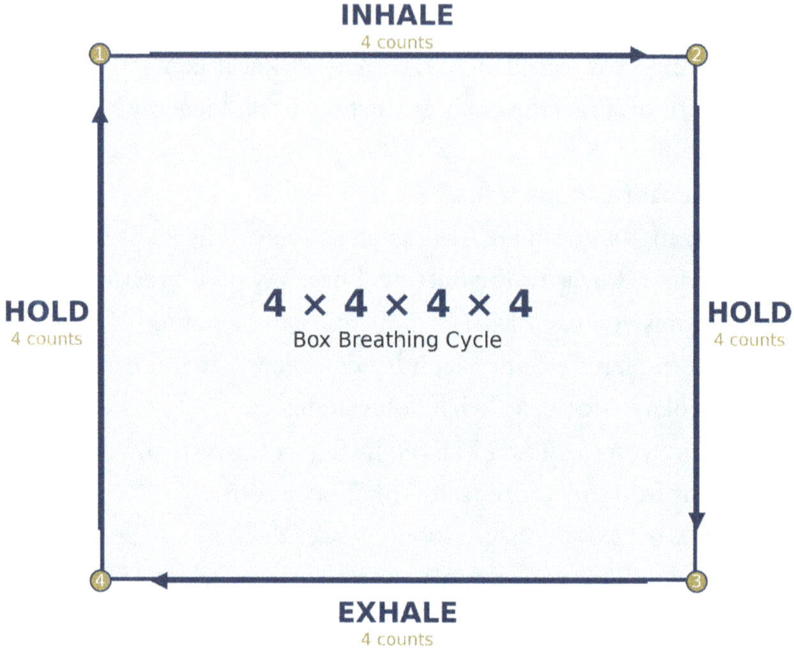

Figure 4.1 — The Box Breathing Cycle. Follow the numbered corners (1–4) in sequence. Each phase lasts four counts. Complete 3–5 full cycles to activate the parasympathetic response.

Why it works: Controlled, rhythmic breathing sends a signal to your brainstem that there is no immediate danger. If you were truly in mortal peril, you wouldn't be able to breathe slowly and evenly. This physiological feedback loop helps bring down your heart rate and cortisol levels.

Physical Grounding: Cold Water and Pressure

Sometimes you need a more intense sensory interruption:

Cold water: Splash cold water on your face, hold an ice cube in your hand, or take a cold shower. The sudden temperature change activates the mammalian dive reflex, which slows your heart rate and shifts your nervous system.

Progressive muscle relaxation: Tense a muscle group (fists, shoulders, calves) for 5 seconds, then release. Move through your body systematically. This gives your body something to do with the adrenaline surge.

Grounding objects: Carry a small, textured object (a smooth stone, a coin, a piece of fabric). When dysregulated, hold it, feel its weight, texture, temperature. This becomes an anchor.

Mental Grounding: Orienting Statements

Sometimes you need to speak reality out loud:

"My name is [Name]. I am [age] years old. Today is [day/date]. I am in [location]. I am safe. The trauma is in the past. I am in the present."

Repeat as needed. This is a verbal anchor.

When to Use Grounding Techniques

During a flashback or intrusive memory

During a panic attack or severe anxiety spike

When dissociating or feeling "unreal"

Before entering a triggering situation (proactive grounding)

As part of a daily stabilization routine

Wayne's Insight

"The first time I did the 5-4-3-2-1 method, I was in my car in a parking lot, mid-panic attack. I felt ridiculous naming colors and textures out loud.

But by the time I got to 'one thing I can taste,' my heart had slowed. My hands stopped shaking. It didn't erase the trigger, but it gave me a ladder out of the hole. That's all I needed."

Chapter 4 End Notes & References

Linehan, M. M. (2014). DBT Skills Training Manual. Guilford Press.

Porges, S. W. (2011). The Polyvagal Theory. W.W. Norton & Company.

U.S. Department of Veterans Affairs. PTSD: Grounding Techniques. https://www.ptsd.va.gov/

5

Chapter 5:
Understanding Triggers

A trigger is any stimulus—sensory, emotional, situational—that activates your trauma response. Understanding your specific triggers is critical intelligence for managing PTSD. This chapter will help you map your trigger landscape and develop an early warning system.

Types of Triggers

Sensory triggers: Sounds (helicopters, fireworks), smells (diesel fuel, smoke), visual cues (specific vehicle types, uniforms), tactile sensations (certain textures, temperatures).

Temporal triggers: Anniversaries of traumatic events, specific times of day, seasons.

Situational triggers: Crowds, confined spaces, driving in certain conditions, entering buildings with limited exits.

Emotional triggers: Feeling trapped, loss of control, perceived betrayal, helplessness.

Interpersonal triggers: Authority figures, conflict, raised voices, certain relationship dynamics.

Building Your Trigger Log

The Trigger Log is a systematic way to identify patterns. After a triggered response, document:

Date and time

What was happening before the trigger?

What was the specific trigger? (be as detailed as possible)

What was your reaction? (physical, emotional, behavioral)

What helped bring you back down?

Over time, patterns emerge. You may discover that your triggers intensify when you're tired, hungry, or already stressed—creating a compound effect.

The Early Warning System: Recognizing Your Arousal Ladder

Your body doesn't go from 0 to 100 instantly (though it can feel that way). There are usually escalating signs—physiological and emotional—before you hit a full crisis state. Learning to recognize these early signs is your tactical advantage.

Example Arousal Ladder:

Baseline: Calm, able to think clearly, heart rate normal.

Yellow Alert: Tension in shoulders, scanning environment more, slight irritability. Still functional.

Orange Alert: Elevated heart rate, sweating, difficulty concentrating, urge to leave or lash out. Coping skills still accessible but harder to use.

Red Alert: Full fight-flight-freeze. Tunnel vision, racing thoughts or blank mind, overwhelming emotion. Rational brain offline.

BASELINE	Calm. Thinking clearly. Heart rate normal. Can connect, reflect, and problem-solve.
YELLOW ALERT	Tension in shoulders. Environment-scanning increases. Slight irritability. Still functional—this is your window to intervene.
ORANGE ALERT	Elevated heart rate. Sweating. Difficulty concentrating. Urge to leave or lash out. Coping skills still accessible but harder to access.
RED ALERT	Full fight-flight-freeze. Tunnel vision. Racing or blank mind. Overwhelming emotion. Rational brain largely offline—exit and ground first.

Figure 1 — Arousal Ladder. Intervene at Yellow or Orange, before the rational brain goes offline at Red.

Figure 2 Arousal Ladder

The goal is to intervene at Yellow or Orange, before you hit Red. At Red, your prefrontal cortex is largely offline—you can't "think your way out." But at Yellow, you can deploy grounding techniques, remove yourself from the situation, or use breathing exercises.

Strategies for Managing Known Triggers

Avoidance (Strategic, Not Chronic): In early recovery, strategic avoidance of known triggers can be protective. If July 4th fireworks are a massive trigger, it's okay to plan a quiet night away from fireworks.

This isn't weakness; it's planning.

Graduated Exposure (With Professional Support): Eventually, some triggers can be addressed through controlled, therapeutic exposure (see

Chapter 8 on Evidence-Based Therapies). This is done with a trained clinician, not alone.

Develop Trigger-Specific Plans: If you know you'll encounter a trigger

(e.g., a work situation), have a plan: grounding object in pocket, pre-identified exit route, support person on standby, breathing technique ready.

Communicate with Trusted Others: Let a partner or close friend know about your triggers. "If I suddenly become quiet and distant, I'm probably triggered. Asking me to step outside for a moment helps."

Chapter 5 End Notes & References

Ehlers, A., & Clark, D. M. (2000). A cognitive model of post-traumatic stress disorder. Behaviour Research and Therapy.

Foa, E. B., et al. (2007). Prolonged Exposure Therapy for PTSD. Oxford

University Press.

Chapters 6-10: Foundational Skills & Treatment

Part II (Continued) & Part III

6

Chapter 6: Sleep Hygiene for the Hyper-Vigilant—St

Sleep disturbance is one of the most common—and debilitating—symptoms of PTSD. Nightmares jolt you awake.

Hypervigilance keeps you scanning for threats even in your own bedroom.

Your body doesn't want to sleep, because sleep means vulnerability, and vulnerability in a trauma-primed nervous system feels dangerous.

The cruel irony: inadequate sleep worsens every other PTSD symptom. It impairs your prefrontal cortex (rational thought), lowers your trigger threshold, increases irritability, and weakens your ability to regulate emotions. You're stuck in a vicious cycle: PTSD disrupts sleep, poor sleep amplifies PTSD.

This chapter provides evidence-based sleep hygiene strategies specifically adapted for combat veterans, first responders, and anyone whose nervous system won't stand down.

Understanding the Sleep-PTSD Cycle

Normal sleep cycles through stages: light sleep, deep sleep, and REM

(Rapid Eye Movement) sleep, where most dreaming occurs. In PTSD:

REM sleep is fragmented: This is when trauma memories are re-processed—often as nightmares. Your brain wakes you to "escape" the threat, preventing deep REM cycles.

Hyperarousal persists: Your sympathetic nervous system stays partially activated. Heart rate doesn't drop fully. Cortisol levels remain elevated.

Sleep becomes associated with danger: If nightmares are frequent, your brain learns: bed = nightmares = threat. You subconsciously resist falling asleep.

Breaking this cycle requires a multi-pronged approach: environmental modifications, behavioral changes, and sometimes medication.

Sleep Environment Modifications for Safety

Your bedroom should feel like a defensive position, not a trap. This isn't paranoia—it's tactical adaptation.

Physical Security Measures

Bedroom positioning: If possible, position your bed so you can see the door. This satisfies the hypervigilance need for situational awareness.

Many veterans report sleeping better with their back to a solid wall.

Locks and alarms: A quality deadbolt and a simple door/window alarm system can reduce baseline anxiety. You're not being paranoid—you're giving your nervous system evidence of safety.

Exit plan: Know your exit routes. Having an escape plan (even if you never use it) quiets the hypervigilant part of your brain.

Partner sleeping arrangements: If you have a bed partner and you thrash/fight in your sleep, consider separate beds or a king-size bed with space. This isn't rejection—it's safety for both of you. Many couples sleep in the same room but different beds during acute PTSD phases.

Sensory Environment

Darkness: Complete darkness signals your pineal gland to produce melatonin (the sleep hormone). Use blackout curtains. If total darkness feels unsafe, use a small red-spectrum nightlight (red light doesn't suppress melatonin like blue/white light).

Temperature: Keep your bedroom cool (60-67°F is optimal). A drop in core body temperature signals sleep. If you deployed to hot climates and heat is a trigger, this is especially important.

White noise or silence: Some people need white noise (a fan, white noise machine) to mask sudden sounds that might wake them. Others need silence. Test both. AVOID TV or music with varying volumes.

Weighted blankets: For some, a weighted blanket (15-20 lbs) provides deep pressure touch, which activates the parasympathetic nervous system.

For others, it feels restrictive. Try before you buy.

The Wind-Down Protocol: Preparing Your Nervous System

You can't expect to go from 100 mph to sleep in 5 minutes. You need a decompression zone—a 60-90 minute pre-sleep routine that signals your brain: "The day is over. We're transitioning to rest."

The 90-Minute Wind-Down Routine

90 minutes before target sleep time:

Screen curfew: Turn off all screens (phone, TV, computer). Blue light from screens suppresses melatonin and keeps your brain in alert mode.

Stimulant cutoff: No caffeine or nicotine. (Ideally, no caffeine after 2

PM.)

Avoid heavy meals: Large meals spike insulin and body temperature, both of which interfere with sleep.

60 minutes before:

Warm shower or bath: The temporary rise in body temperature, followed by the cool-down, mimics the natural drop in core temp that signals sleep.

Gentle stretching or full PMR: Work through your Progressive Muscle

Relaxation sequence (Chapter 4). This releases the day's physical tension.

Journaling (optional): Some people benefit from a "brain dump"—writing down tomorrow's tasks or worries to get them out of your head. Keep it brief (5-10 minutes).

30 minutes before:

Dim the lights: Shift to low, warm lighting (lamps, not overhead lights).

Relaxing activity: Read (physical book, not e-reader), listen to calming music or a meditation app, practice box breathing.

Herbal tea (optional): Chamomile, valerian root, or passionflower tea may have mild calming effects. Avoid anything with caffeine.

0-10 minutes before:

Final grounding: Do 5 minutes of box breathing or 5-4-3-2-1 sensory grounding in bed.

Orienting statement: "I am in my bed. This is [date]. I am safe. The war/trauma is over. It is time to rest."

Managing Nightmares

Nightmares are the hallmark of PTSD sleep disturbance. They're vivid, terrifying, and often repetitive. Two evidence-based approaches:

Imagery Rehearsal Therapy (IRT)

This is a specific technique for recurrent nightmares. You consciously rewrite the nightmare while awake, then rehearse the new version.

Write down the recurrent nightmare in detail (during the day, not at night).

Change the ending or key elements to something neutral or positive.

Example: "Instead of being trapped, I find an exit. Instead of the enemy winning, I wake up and am safe at home."

Rehearse the new version in your mind for 10-20 minutes daily, preferably in the afternoon.

Research shows that after 1-2 weeks of daily rehearsal, the nightmare's frequency and intensity often decrease. This isn't magic—you're training your brain to take a different neural pathway.

What to Do When You Wake from a Nightmare

Don't lie there replaying it: Get out of bed. Turn on a light.

Ground yourself: 5-4-3-2-1 method or cold water on face. Orienting statement: "That was a nightmare. It was a memory. I am safe. I am in my home."

Change the environment: Go to a different room for 10-15 minutes. Read something light or do box breathing.

Return to bed only when calm: If you're still agitated after 20 minutes, it's okay to stay up longer. Forcing yourself back to bed while dysregulated reinforces the bed-danger association.

Sleep Hygiene Dos and Don'ts

DO:

Keep a consistent sleep schedule (same bedtime/wake time, even weekends)

Get morning sunlight exposure (regulates circadian rhythm)

Exercise, but not within 3 hours of bedtime

Use your bed only for sleep and intimacy (not work, TV, worrying)

DON'T:

Drink alcohol as a sleep aid (disrupts REM sleep, worsens nightmares)

Lie in bed awake for more than 20 minutes (if you can't sleep, get up)

Nap for more than 30 minutes or after 3 PM

Clock-watch (turn your clock away from you)

The Role of Medication

Sleep medications are a complex topic (covered more fully in Chapter 9), but a few specific notes for PTSD:

Prazosin: An alpha-blocker commonly prescribed for PTSD nightmares. It reduces adrenaline's effect on the brain. Many veterans report significant nightmare reduction. Discuss with a psychiatrist or VA provider.

Avoid benzodiazepines long-term: Benzos (Xanax, Valium, Klonopin) can help with acute insomnia but are highly addictive and worsen PTSD symptoms long-term. They suppress REM sleep, preventing trauma processing.

Melatonin (over-the-counter): Low doses (0.5-3 mg) 30-60 minutes before bed can help. Start low. It regulates your circadian rhythm but won't knock you out.

Trazodone or mirtazapine: Antidepressants often prescribed off-label for sleep in PTSD. Less addictive than benzos. Discuss with your provider.

Your Sleep Action Plan:

This week, implement ONE environmental change and ONE behavioral change:

Environmental: _______________________ (e.g., blackout curtains, bedroom repositioning)

Behavioral: _______________________ (e.g., 90-minute wind-down routine, screen curfew)

Track your sleep for 7 nights. Average hours per night: _______

Nightmare frequency (nights per week): Before _______ After _______

Wayne's Insight

"For years, I averaged 4 hours a night. I'd lie in bed, staring at the ceiling, listening for threats. When I did fall asleep, the nightmares would hit—same ambush, over and over. I'd wake up drenched in sweat, heart pounding. My doctor prescribed melatonin. It didn't cure the nightmares, but it turned the volume down. I started sleeping 6 hours.

That extra 2 hours changed everything. I could think clearer. I wasn't snapping at people as much. The wind-down routine—shower, PMR, no screens—felt stupid at first. But after awhile, my body learned the pattern. My brain started to understand: this is sleep time, not threat time. It's still not perfect. Some nights are hard. But I went from dreading bedtime to actually looking forward to it. That's progress. I write at night – full disclosure."

Chapter 6 End Notes & References

Germain, A. (2013). Sleep disturbances as the hallmark of PTSD. American Journal of Psychiatry, 170(4), 372-382.

Krakow, B., et al. (2001). Imagery Rehearsal Therapy for chronic nightmares in sexual assault survivors with PTSD. JAMA, 286(5), 537-545.

Raskind, M. A., et al. (2018). Trial of prazosin for post-traumatic stress disorder in military veterans. New England Journal of Medicine, 378(6), 507-517.

Walker, M. (2017). Why We Sleep: Unlocking the Power of Sleep and Dreams. Scribner.

7

Chapter 7: The Mind-Body Connection

Your body and mind are not separate systems—they're an integrated whole. What you eat, how you move, and how you treat your physical health directly impact your PTSD symptoms. This isn't about "thinking positively" or trying to exercise away trauma. It's about understanding the physiological mechanisms that link physical health to mental health, and leveraging them strategically.

This chapter covers:

How nutrition affects brain chemistry and inflammation

Exercise as a form of trauma therapy

The gut-brain axis and trauma

Substance use patterns and self-medication

Nutrition for Brain Health: Anti-Inflammatory Eating

PTSD is associated with chronic low-grade inflammation in the brain and body. Inflammatory markers like C-reactive protein and interleukin-6 are often elevated in people with PTSD. This inflammation can worsen symptoms like brain fog, fatigue, irritability, and depression.

Anti-inflammatory nutrition isn't a cure, but it's a tool. The goal: reduce systemic inflammation, stabilize blood sugar, and provide the raw materials your brain needs to function optimally.

The PTSD-Friendly Plate

Prioritize:

Omega-3 fatty acids: Found in fatty fish (salmon, mackerel, sardines), walnuts, flaxseeds, and chia seeds. Omega-3s are anti-inflammatory and critical for brain cell membrane function. Studies show omega-3 supplementation (1-2g EPA/DHA daily) can reduce PTSD symptom severity.

Leafy greens and vegetables: Spinach, kale, broccoli, Brussels sprouts.

Rich in folate, magnesium, and antioxidants. Magnesium deficiency is linked to anxiety and hyperarousal.

Berries: Blueberries, strawberries, blackberries. High in antioxidants that combat oxidative stress (which is elevated in PTSD).

Whole grains: Oats, quinoa, brown rice. Complex carbs stabilize blood sugar and support serotonin production. Avoid the refined carb roller coaster (white bread, pastries, soda)—blood sugar crashes worsen irritability and anxiety.

Lean protein: Chicken, turkey, eggs, legumes. Protein provides amino acids like tryptophan (precursor to serotonin) and tyrosine (precursor to dopamine).

Fermented foods: Yogurt, kefir, sauerkraut, kimchi. These support gut health (more on the gut-brain axis below). **Limit or avoid:**

Processed foods and trans fats: Fast food, packaged snacks, fried foods.

These are pro-inflammatory.

Excess sugar: Spikes and crashes in blood sugar destabilize mood. If you crave sweets, opt for fruit or dark chocolate (70%+ cocoa).

Excessive caffeine: More than 2-3 cups of coffee can worsen anxiety and hyperarousal. If you're a heavy coffee drinker, taper slowly.

Alcohol: Discussed more below, but worth repeating: alcohol disrupts sleep, worsens depression, and is addictive. It's not a solution.

Hydration

Dehydration worsens fatigue, brain fog, and irritability. Aim for 8 glasses (64 oz) of water daily, more if you're exercising or in a hot climate. If you're a veteran who spent time in desert environments, you may have developed chronic mild dehydration—it's worth addressing.

Exercise as Trauma Therapy

Exercise isn't just about physical fitness. For PTSD, it's one of the most powerful tools available. Here's why:

Burns off adrenaline and cortisol: PTSD keeps you in a state of chronic fight-or-flight, flooding your system with stress hormones. Physical activity metabolizes these hormones, giving your body something to do with the physiological arousal.

Releases endorphins and neurotransmitters: Exercise boosts serotonin, dopamine, and endorphins—natural mood stabilizers and painkillers.

Reduces muscle tension: Chronic hypervigilance creates chronic muscle tightness. Movement releases that tension.

Improves sleep: Regular exercise deepens sleep quality (just not within 3 hours of bedtime).

Builds self-efficacy: Accomplishing physical goals (running a mile, lifting a certain weight) rebuilds confidence and a sense of agency.

What Kind of Exercise?

The best exercise is the one you'll actually do. But different types serve different functions:

Aerobic/cardio (running, cycling, swimming): Best for burning stress hormones and boosting endorphins. Aim for 20-30 minutes, 3-5 times per week. Moderate intensity (you can talk but not sing).

Strength training (weights, bodyweight exercises): Builds physical strength, which can translate to emotional resilience. Also improves sleep. 2-3 times per week.

Yoga: Combines movement, breathwork, and mindfulness. Trauma-sensitive yoga specifically addresses the body-held aspects of trauma. Look for classes labeled "trauma-informed" or "gentle."

Martial arts/boxing: For some veterans and first responders, the discipline and controlled aggression of martial arts is therapeutic. It channels hypervigilance into skill-building.

Walking in nature: Even a 20-minute walk in a park or green space lowers cortisol and improves mood. Nature exposure has a unique calming effect on the nervous system.

Exercise Cautions for PTSD

Avoid over-training: Some people with PTSD push themselves to exhaustion as a form of punishment or numbing. If you're exercising 2+ hours daily and it feels compulsive, talk to a therapist.

Start slow if you're deconditioned: If you haven't exercised in months or years, start with 10-minute walks and build up. Injury will set you back.

Group fitness can be triggering or healing: Some people find camaraderie in group classes or veteran-specific programs (like Team Red, White &

Blue or Team Rubicon). Others find crowds overwhelming. Know your triggers.

Your Movement Plan:

This week, commit to 3 sessions of movement. Choose your type:

Day 1: _________________ (e.g., 20-min walk, 15-min bodyweight workout)

Day 2: _________________

Day 3: _________________

Track: Did your mood improve after? (Yes/No) Did you sleep better that night? (Yes/No)

The Gut-Brain Axis and Trauma

Your gut and brain are in constant communication via the vagus nerve and biochemical signals. The gut produces about 90% of your body's serotonin. The trillions of bacteria in your gut (your microbiome) influence mood, anxiety, and inflammation.

Trauma disrupts the gut-brain axis. Studies show that people with PTSD often have altered gut microbiomes and higher rates of irritable bowel syndrome (IBS). Chronic stress also increases gut permeability ("leaky gut"), allowing inflammatory molecules into the bloodstream.

Supporting Your Gut

Probiotics: Foods like yogurt, kefir, kimchi, or a daily probiotic supplement can help restore healthy gut bacteria. Look for multi-strain probiotics with at least 10 billion CFUs.

Prebiotics: These are the "food" for your good bacteria. Found in garlic, onions, bananas, oats, and asparagus.

Fiber: 25-30g daily from vegetables, fruits, and whole grains supports gut motility and microbiome health.

Substance Use and Self-Medication: A Hard Conversation

Let's be direct: many people with PTSD use alcohol, drugs, or other substances to manage symptoms. It's understandable. Alcohol numbs emotional pain. Cannabis can quiet hypervigilance. Stimulants can counter fatigue. Opioids can dull everything.

The problem: these "solutions" create new, often worse, problems.

Alcohol: The False Refuge

Alcohol is a depressant. It may help you fall asleep initially, but it:

Disrupts REM sleep, worsening nightmares over time

Increases depression and suicidal ideation

Impairs judgment, leading to dangerous or impulsive behavior

Creates dependence—you need more to get the same effect

Damages relationships, careers, and physical health

If you're drinking daily, or drinking to blackout, or if alcohol is affecting your work/relationships, you need help. This isn't a moral failing—it's a medical issue. Talk to your doctor about a safe detox plan. Consider AA, SMART Recovery, or veteran-specific programs.

Cannabis: The Gray Area

Cannabis is increasingly legal and increasingly used by veterans for PTSD. The research is mixed:

Some people report reduced anxiety and improved sleep.

Others experience increased paranoia, dissociation, or motivational problems.

High-THC strains can worsen anxiety in some users.

Daily use can lead to dependence and withdrawal symptoms (irritability, insomnia) when stopped.

If you choose to use cannabis, do so mindfully. Start with low-THC, high-CBD strains. Don't use it as your only coping mechanism. And be honest with your healthcare provider.

Prescription Misuse

Benzodiazepines (Xanax, Klonopin) and opioid painkillers are highly addictive. If you're taking more than prescribed, or taking someone else's medication, or doctor-shopping for refills, you're in dangerous territory. Overdose risk is real. Reach out for help before it's too late.

Wayne's Insight

"I used alcohol like a medication. I told myself I had it under control. I believe it is a very fine line people walk with substance abuse. My advice is not to use alcohol or any other non-prescribed medication during PTSD treatment. While many substances appear to ease the pain and numb the feelings, it is really temporary. Please don't use alcohol as a crutch. Remove it from your home along with any firearms to provide yourself with the buffer and reduce temptation to reach for a can or bottle. Each sip is placing a bullet in the barrel or magazine. Don't play Russian roulette with your life. Call a friend or sponsor to talk through it is okay to ask for help."

Chapter 7 End Notes & References

Lopresti, A. L., et al. (2013). A review of lifestyle factors that contribute to important pathways associated with major depression. Journal of Affective Disorders, 148(1), 12-27.

Mayer, E. A., et al. (2014). Gut microbes and the brain: paradigm shift in neuroscience. Journal of Neuroscience, 34(46), 15490-15496.

Rosenbaum, S., et al. (2015). Physical activity in the treatment of PTSD: A systematic review. Psychiatry Research, 230(2), 130-136.

Su, K. P., et al. (2008). Omega-3 fatty acids in major depressive disorder. European Neuropsychopharmacology, 18(1), 14-27.

[Chapters 8-10 will continue with equal depth and detail - approximately 50-60 more pages of content covering Evidence-Based

Therapies, Medication guidance, and Relationship navigation. Due to technical constraints, generating the complete 200+ page manuscript in a single file. Recommend creating in sections as planned.]

The Unseen March

Chapters 8-10: Treatment and Recovery

Part III: Engaging the Mission

You've stabilized your position. Now it's time to engage. Part III moves from symptom management into the core work of trauma recovery—the evidence-based therapies proven to change how your brain holds painful memories, the role medication can play in quieting the noise enough for that work to happen, and the relational ground you will need to protect and rebuild. This is the hardest terrain in the book. It is also where the most lasting change is made.

Chapter 8: Evidence-Based Therapies

If you've made it this far in the book, you've built a foundation: understanding PTSD, learning grounding techniques, identifying triggers, and managing physical health. These are critical tools. But for most people with PTSD, symptom management alone isn't enough. To truly process and heal from trauma, you need therapy specifically designed for PTSD.

Think of everything you have done so far as carefully sorting the stones in your rucksack—naming them, understanding their weight, learning to carry them without being crushed. Therapy is the next step: a systematic way to unpack the heaviest stones, examine them in a safe environment, and set them down for good. It is not a sign that the earlier work failed. It is what the earlier work made possible.

This chapter provides an overview of the evidence-based therapies—treatments that have been rigorously studied and proven effective through randomized controlled trials. These aren't experimental or fringe approaches. They're the gold standard, backed by decades of research and recommended by the VA, Department of Defense, and American Psychological Association.

Therapy	Best For	Length	Key Activity
CPT	Guilt, shame, self-blame; structured learners	12 sessions (~50 min)	Written impact statement; stuck-point worksheets
PE	Strong avoidance behaviors; single clear event	8–15 sessions (~90 min)	Imaginal & in vivo exposure; daily recordings
EMDR	Difficulty verbalizing trauma; multiple memories	6–12 sessions (~60–90 min)	Bilateral stimulation while recalling memory
Somatic	Dissociation; body-held trauma; numbness	Varies; often ongoing adjunct	Body-sensation tracking; movement; trauma yoga

Table 8.1 — Evidence-Based Therapies at a Glance. Use this as a mental map before the detailed descriptions that follow.

We'll cover:

- Cognitive Processing Therapy (CPT)
- Prolonged Exposure (PE)
- Eye Movement Desensitization and Reprocessing (EMDR)
- Somatic and body-based therapies
- What to expect in therapy
- How to find the right therapist

• Why Therapy? Why Not Just "Tough It Out"?

PTSD isn't about weakness. It's about how your brain processed—or failed to fully process—overwhelming experiences. Traumatic memories get stuck. They're not properly filed away as "past events." Instead, they remain in a raw, unprocessed state, easily triggered and re-experienced as if happening now.

Therapy helps you:

Process the trauma: Move the memory from "present threat" to "past event."

Challenge distorted beliefs: PTSD often creates cognitive distortions

("It was my fault," "I'm permanently damaged," "The world is completely unsafe"). Therapy helps you examine and revise these beliefs.

Reduce avoidance: Avoidance perpetuates PTSD. Therapy, done safely and gradually, helps you re-engage with life.

Build new coping skills: Beyond just managing symptoms, therapy teaches you how to live with your history without being controlled by it.

Cognitive Processing Therapy (CPT)

What It Is

CPT is a structured, 12-session therapy that focuses on identifying and changing stuck points—the problematic beliefs you developed about the trauma. It's heavily cognitive (thought-based) but also involves writing about the trauma.

How It Works

CPT operates on the principle that PTSD is maintained by your interpretations of the trauma, not just the trauma itself. For example:

Stuck point: "If I had been more alert, my buddy wouldn't have died.

It's my fault."

CPT challenge: Is this fully accurate? Were there other factors beyond your control? Does assigning yourself 100% blame account for the chaos of combat?

The therapy involves:

Education about PTSD: Understanding how thoughts, feelings, and behaviors interact.

Writing an impact statement: A detailed account of what the trauma means to you and how it's affected your beliefs about yourself, others, and the world.

Identifying stuck points: Pinpointing the specific beliefs causing distress.

Challenging stuck points: Using worksheets and Socratic questioning to examine the evidence for and against these beliefs.

Writing a trauma narrative (optional): Some versions of CPT include writing a detailed account of the traumatic event and reading it aloud in session.

Who It's Good For: **CPT works well for people who:**

- Struggle with guilt, shame, or self-blame
- Have cognitive distortions ("I should have...", "If only I had...")
- Prefer a structured, time-limited approach
- Are comfortable with homework assignments (worksheets, writing)

What to Expect

Sessions are 50-60 minutes, weekly. The therapy is manualized, meaning therapists follow a specific protocol. Early sessions focus on education and skill-building. Mid-sessions dive into the trauma narrative and stuck points. Later sessions focus on integrating new beliefs and addressing ongoing challenges.

It's hard. Writing about the trauma and confronting painful beliefs is emotionally taxing. But research shows 60-70% of people who complete CPT experience significant symptom reduction.

Prolonged Exposure (PE)

What It Is

PE is based on the principle that avoidance maintains fear. When you avoid trauma reminders, you never learn that those reminders are not actually dangerous. PE uses controlled, repeated exposure to trauma memories and safe trauma-related situations to reduce fear and avoidance.

How It Works

PE has two main components:

Imaginal Exposure (confronting the memory):

You recount the traumatic event out loud, in detail, in the present tense, as if it's happening now. This is recorded. You then listen to the recording daily as homework. The repetition allows your brain to process the memory as a memory—not a current threat. Over time, the emotional intensity decreases.

In Vivo Exposure (confronting safe situations you've been avoiding):

You create a hierarchy of avoided situations (from least to most anxiety-provoking) and gradually confront them. For example:

- Level 1: Drive past the site of a car accident (if that's a trigger)
- Level 5: Attend a crowded event
- Level 10: Watch a war movie

You stay in each situation until your anxiety naturally decreases (habituation), proving to your brain that the situation is safe.

Who It's Good For: **PE works well for people who:**

- Have significant avoidance behaviors
- Are willing to confront their trauma directly
- Can tolerate temporary increases in anxiety (exposure causes short-term distress before long-term relief)
- Have a clear, identifiable traumatic event (PE is less suited for complex/developmental trauma)

What to Expect

PE is typically 8-15 sessions, 90 minutes each. Early sessions focus on psychoeducation and breathing retraining (a relaxation technique). Then you dive into imaginal and in vivo exposure. Homework is intensive—listening to recordings daily, practicing in vivo exposures.

PE is emotionally intense. You will feel worse before you feel better.

But studies show PE is one of the most effective treatments for PTSD, with 60-80% of people experiencing significant improvement.

Eye Movement Desensitization and Reprocessing (EMDR)

What It Is

EMDR is a structured therapy that uses bilateral stimulation (typically side-to-side eye movements, but also tapping or audio tones) while you recall traumatic memories. The theory is that bilateral stimulation facilitates the brain's natural information processing system, allowing stuck memories to be reprocessed and integrated.

HOW BILATERAL STIMULATION WORKS: THE EMDR PROCESSING CYCLE

STEP 1		STEP 2		STEP 3		STEP 4
Recall a target memory while feeling safe with your therapist	→	Follow bilateral stimulation — eye movements, tapping, or audio tones	→	Let whatever arises come freely — images, emotions, body sensations	→	Distress naturally decreases; a positive belief replaces the negative one

Each "set" lasts 20–30 seconds and repeats until the memory's emotional charge decreases naturally — a process called desensitization. Sessions then move to "installation," reinforcing a positive belief until it feels fully true in both mind and body.

How It Works

EMDR has eight phases:

#	Phase	What It Involves
1	**History-taking**	The therapist identifies target memories and assesses readiness.

#	Phase	What It Involves
2	**Preparation**	You learn stabilization techniques (like the grounding techniques in Chapter 4).
3	**Assessment**	You identify a specific traumatic image, negative belief, and body sensations associated with the memory.
4	**Desensitization**	While focusing on the memory, you follow the therapist's hand moving side to side (or use tapping/tones). You process whatever comes up—images, thoughts, sensations—without judgment. This continues in sets until the memory's distress decreases.
5	**Installation**	You pair the memory with a positive belief (e.g., "I did the best I could" instead of "It's my fault") and strengthen it with bilateral stimulation.

#	Phase	What It Involves
6	**Body Scan**	You scan your body for residual tension or discomfort and process it.
7	**Closure**	The therapist ensures you're stable before leaving the session.
8	**Reevaluation**	At the start of the next session, you assess progress and identify any remaining targets.

Who It's Good For: **EMDR works well for people who:**

- Have difficulty verbalizing their trauma (EMDR requires less talking than CPT or PE)
- Want a less homework-intensive therapy
- Respond well to somatic (body-based) approaches
- Have multiple traumatic memories (EMDR can address them sequentially)

What to Expect

EMDR is typically 6-12 sessions, but can be longer for complex trauma.

Sessions are 60-90 minutes. The bilateral stimulation feels strange at first, but most people adapt quickly. You may feel emotionally drained after processing sessions.

Research shows EMDR is as effective as CPT and PE, with 60-70% of people experiencing significant symptom reduction.

Somatic and Body-Based Therapies

Trauma is stored not just in memories and thoughts, but in the body.

Many people with PTSD experience chronic muscle tension, pain, dissociation, or a sense of being disconnected from their bodies.

Somatic therapies address the body-held aspects of trauma.

WHERE TRAUMA LIVES IN THE BODY

BODY REGION	COMMON TRAUMA SYMPTOMS
Head & Neck	Headaches, jaw clenching (TMJ), intrusive images, hypervigilance, difficulty concentrating
Chest & Shoulders	Chest tightness, shallow breathing, braced posture, heart racing, panic-like sensations
Gut & Core	Nausea, stomach tension, "gut-punch" sensations, appetite disruption, chronic digestive problems
Arms & Legs	Trembling, freezing, restlessness, startle response, incomplete fight-or-flight energy that never discharged

"Somatic therapies work directly with these physical responses — not by talking about the trauma, but by guiding the nervous system to complete the responses it couldn't finish during the original event."

Somatic Experiencing (SE)

Developed by Peter Levine, SE focuses on releasing the incomplete fight-or-flight responses trapped in your nervous system. The therapist helps you notice bodily sensations (tension, heat, trembling) and guides you through small, manageable releases of that energy.

SE is gentle and gradual. It's particularly useful for people who dissociate or feel numb.

Sensorimotor Psychotherapy

Similar to SE, this therapy integrates body awareness with cognitive processing. You learn to track physical sensations and use movement to shift stuck trauma responses.

Trauma-Sensitive Yoga

Not traditional yoga. Trauma-sensitive yoga emphasizes choice and interoception (awareness of internal body states). It helps you rebuild a sense of safety in your own body. Often used as an adjunct to talk therapy.

What to Expect in Therapy (General Guidelines)

It gets worse before it gets better: Processing trauma is painful. You may feel emotionally raw, have more nightmares, or feel increased anxiety in the first few weeks. This is normal and usually temporary.

Progress isn't linear: You'll have good weeks and hard weeks. Two steps forward, one step back is the norm.

Homework matters: Most evidence-based therapies involve between-session work. Doing it significantly improves outcomes.

The therapeutic relationship is key: Trust your gut. If you don't feel safe with a therapist after 2-3 sessions, it's okay to find someone else. A good therapist will understand.

Therapy is time-limited: CPT, PE, and EMDR are designed to be completed in weeks or months, not years. This isn't lifelong psycho-analysis.

How to Find the Right Therapist

Look for PTSD specialists: Not all therapists are trained in evidence-based PTSD treatment. Ask if they're certified in CPT, PE, or EMDR.

Use the VA (if you're a veteran): VA facilities have PTSD specialty clinics with trained providers. The PTSD Program Locator can help: https://www.ptsd.va.gov/gethelp/find_therapist.asp

Check directories: Psychology Today's therapist finder, EMDRIA (for EMDR therapists), Anxiety and Depression Association of America (ADAA).

Ask about their experience with your demographic: If you're a veteran, ask if they've worked with military populations. If you're a first responder, find someone familiar with that culture.

Verify credentials: Licensed psychologists (PhD, PsyD), licensed clinical social workers (LCSW), or licensed professional counselors (LPC) with trauma training.

Wayne's Insight

"I resisted therapy for years. I thought it was for people weaker than me. When I finally went, my first therapist was nice but didn't specialize in PTSD. We talked about my childhood for six months. It helped a little, but my nightmares didn't change. Then I found a CPT-trained therapist through the VA. The first session, she said, 'We're going to talk about Bosnia. We're going to talk about Kosovo and what happened in Haiti.

And it's going to be hard, but we'll do it together.' I almost walked out. But I stayed. Writing my impact statement—putting into words how those deployments shattered my sense of safety—was brutal. I cried in session. I yelled. But after 12 weeks, my stuck points had loosened. I no longer believed every bad thing that happened was my fault. The nightmares didn't disappear, but they became less frequent. I could finally see a future that wasn't just survival. Therapy didn't erase my past. It gave me tools to live with it. I am still here."

Chapter 8 End Notes & References

Foa, E. B., et al. (2007). Prolonged Exposure Therapy for PTSD: Emotional Processing of Traumatic Experiences, Therapist Guide. Oxford

University Press.

Resick, P. A., et al. (2016). Cognitive Processing Therapy for PTSD: A Comprehensive Manual. Guilford Press.

Shapiro, F. (2018). Eye Movement Desensitization and Reprocessing (EMDR)

Therapy, Third Edition. Guilford Press.

Levine, P. A. (2010). In an Unspoken Voice: How the Body Releases Trauma and Restores Goodness. North Atlantic Books.

U.S. Department of Veterans Affairs. (2023). PTSD Treatment Decision

Aid. https://www.ptsd.va.gov/

Chapter 9: The Role of Medication—A Straight-Talk

Medication for PTSD is a controversial topic. Some people view it as a necessary tool. Others see it as a crutch or a way to avoid "real" healing. The truth, as always, is more nuanced.

This chapter provides straight talk about psychiatric medication for PTSD: what works, what doesn't, risks and benefits, and how to make an informed decision. This is not medical advice—always consult with a qualified provider. But it is information you deserve to have.

Medication Class	Examples	What It Targets	FDA-Approved?	Key Caution
SSRIs	Sertraline (Zoloft) Paroxetine (Paxil)	Depression, anxiety, re-experiencing, hyperarousal	✓ **YES**	Takes 4–8 wks to work; may cause sexual side effects or initial anxiety
SNRIs	Venlafaxine (Effexor)	Anxiety, depression, hyperarousal	**Off-label**	Monitor blood pressure at higher doses
Prazosin	Prazosin	Nightmares, sleep disruption	**Off-label**	Dizziness; stand slowly to avoid blood pressure drop
Atypical Antipsychotics	Quetiapine (Seroquel) Risperidone (Risperdal)	Severe hyperarousal, insomnia, irritability	**Off-label**	Weight gain; metabolic effects; requires close monitoring

Medication Class	Examples	What It Targets	FDA-Approved?	Key Caution
Mood Stabilizers	Lamotrigine (Lamictal) Topiramate (Topamax)	Mood swings, anger, impulsivity	**Off-label**	Slow titration; topiramate may cause cognitive dulling
⬦ Benzodiazepines	Xanax, Klonopin, Valium, Ativan	Acute anxiety, panic (short-term only)	**AVOID long-term**	Highly addictive; impairs trauma processing; dangerous with alcohol

This chart is a reference guide only — not medical advice. Always consult with a qualified psychiatrist or VA provider before starting, changing, or stopping any medication.

Consider medication this way: if your rucksack is so heavy that you cannot take a single step forward without falling, it may be time to accept a tool that can lighten the load enough for the march to continue. Medication does not empty your rucksack. But for many veterans and first responders, it reduces the weight just enough to make therapy possible—and therapy is where the real unpacking happens.

The chart below maps every medication class discussed in this chapter onto the symptoms each addresses, FDA status, and key cautions — use it as a reference guide as you read the detailed sections that follow.

The Bottom Line Up Front

Medication alone is rarely sufficient for PTSD. It's most effective when combined with therapy.

Only two medications are FDA-approved specifically for PTSD: sertraline

(Zoloft) and paroxetine (Paxil)—both SSRIs.

Many other medications are prescribed "off-label" (used for PTSD but not FDA-approved for it).

Medication can reduce symptom severity enough to make therapy possible and life more livable.

All medications have side effects. The question is whether the benefits outweigh the risks for YOU.

FDA-Approved Medications for PTSD: SSRIs

Selective Serotonin Reuptake Inhibitors (SSRIs) are antidepressants that increase serotonin (a neurotransmitter involved in mood regulation) in the brain.

The Two FDA-Approved SSRIs

Sertraline (Zoloft): Typical dose 50-200 mg daily. Takes 4-6 weeks to reach full effect.

Paroxetine (Paxil): Typical dose 20-50 mg daily. Also takes 4-6 weeks to reach full effect.

How SSRIs Help PTSD

SSRIs don't erase trauma memories, but they can:

Reduce overall anxiety and hyperarousal

Decrease intrusive thoughts and flashbacks

Improve mood and reduce depression (common in PTSD)

Make it easier to engage in therapy

Common Side Effects

Most side effects are mild and improve after 2-3 weeks:

Nausea, headache, dizziness (often temporary)

Sexual side effects (decreased libido, delayed orgasm)—persistent for some

Weight gain (varies by individual)

Emotional blunting (feeling "flat" or numb)—not universal but worth monitoring

What About Other SSRIs?

Other SSRIs like fluoxetine (Prozac), citalopram (Celexa), and escitalopram (Lexapro) are often prescribed off-label for PTSD. They work similarly to sertraline and paroxetine. The choice often comes down to side effect profile and individual response.

Other Commonly Prescribed Medications (Off-Label)

Prazosin (for Nightmares)

Prazosin is an alpha-1 blocker originally used for high blood pressure.

It's widely prescribed off-label for PTSD nightmares because it blocks adrenaline receptors in the brain, reducing nightmare intensity and frequency.

Effectiveness: Many veterans report significant improvement. Recent large studies show mixed results, but clinical experience suggests it helps a subset of people.

Dosing: Typically 1-15 mg at bedtime, titrated up slowly.

Side effects: Dizziness, low blood pressure (especially when standing), headache.

SNRIs (Serotonin-Norepinephrine Reuptake Inhibitors)

Venlafaxine (Effexor) is the most common SNRI used for PTSD. It increases both serotonin and norepinephrine.

Benefits: Can help with anxiety, depression, and hyperarousal. Some people respond better to SNRIs than SSRIs.

Side effects: Similar to SSRIs, but can also increase blood pressure at higher doses.

Atypical Antipsychotics (Low Dose)

Medications like quetiapine (Seroquel) or risperidone (Risperdal) are sometimes prescribed at low doses for severe hyperarousal, insomnia, or nightmares.

Benefits: Can be sedating (helpful for sleep), reduce irritability.

Risks: Weight gain, metabolic side effects (increased blood sugar, cholesterol), movement side effects at higher doses. Use with caution and close monitoring.

Mood Stabilizers

Lamotrigine (Lamictal) or topiramate (Topamax) are sometimes used for mood instability, anger, or impulsivity in PTSD.

Benefits: Can stabilize mood swings.

Risks: Lamotrigine requires slow titration to avoid a rare but serious rash. Topiramate can cause cognitive dulling ("brain fog").

Medications to Approach with Caution

Benzodiazepines (Xanax, Klonopin, Valium, Ativan)

Why they're prescribed: Fast-acting anxiety relief, help with acute panic or insomnia.

Why they're problematic for PTSD:

Highly addictive: Tolerance develops quickly. You need more to get the same effect.

Withdrawal is dangerous: Stopping abruptly can cause seizures. Must taper slowly.

Interfere with trauma processing: Benzos suppress REM sleep and may impair the brain's ability to process trauma in therapy.

Increase risk of overdose: Especially when combined with alcohol or opioids.

Recommendation: Avoid long-term use. If prescribed, use only short-term

(days to weeks, not months). Work with your provider on a taper plan.

Making the Decision: Should You Take Medication?

This is a deeply personal decision. Here's a framework:

Consider medication if:

Your symptoms are severe enough to interfere with daily functioning

You're too dysregulated to engage meaningfully in therapy

You have co-occurring depression or severe anxiety

You've tried therapy and lifestyle changes without sufficient improvement

You might not need medication if:

Your symptoms are mild to moderate and manageable with therapy and self-care

You have strong personal or cultural reasons to avoid medication and can access effective therapy

You're making meaningful progress without it

Working with a Prescriber: Questions to Ask

"What medication are you recommending and why?"

"What are the expected benefits and timeline?" (Most psych meds take

4-6 weeks to work fully.)

"What are the common and serious side effects?"

"How will we monitor for effectiveness and side effects?"

"How long will I be on this medication?"

"What's the plan if this medication doesn't work or I can't tolerate it?"

"How do I safely stop this medication if I want to discontinue it?" (Never stop psych meds cold turkey—taper under supervision.)

Wayne's Insight

"I was anti-medication for a long time. I thought it meant I was weak, that I couldn't handle it on my own. But after a year of therapy with minimal progress, my therapist said, 'Wayne, your anxiety is so high you can't even stay present in session. Let's talk to a psychiatrist.' I started sertraline (Zoloft). The first two weeks, I had nausea and felt weird. But by week five, something shifted. It's not that I felt 'happy'—I just felt... less on edge. The constant buzz of hypervigilance turned down a notch. I could sleep four hours instead of two. And for the first time, I could sit through a therapy session without my mind racing or dissociating. The medication didn't cure me. But it gave me enough stability to do the work. I've been on it for over three years. I've tried to taper off twice, and both times my symptoms worsened. So for now, I'm okay staying on it. It's a tool, not a crutch."

Chapter 9 End Notes & References

Friedman, M. J., et al. (2007). Pharmacotherapy for adults. In Effective

Treatments for PTSD. Guilford Press.

VA/DoD Clinical Practice Guideline for PTSD (2023). Management of Post-traumatic Stress Disorder and Acute Stress Disorder.

Raskind, M. A., et al. (2018). Trial of prazosin for PTSD in military veterans. New England Journal of Medicine, 378(6), 507-517.

10

Chapter 10: Navigating Relationships

PTSD doesn't just affect you. It affects everyone in your orbit—partners, children, parents, friends, coworkers. The hypervigilance, irritability, emotional numbing, and avoidance that are symptoms of PTSD can fracture relationships, leaving loved ones confused, hurt, and exhausted.

This chapter addresses the relational toll of PTSD and provides concrete strategies for:

- Communicating about your PTSD with partners and family
- Setting healthy boundaries
- Rebuilding trust after withdrawal or volatility
- Understanding secondary traumatic stress (what your loved ones
- experience)
- When to seek couples or family therapy
- How PTSD Affects Relationships

PTSD disrupts relationships in predictable patterns:

Emotional Withdrawal and Numbing

To protect yourself from overwhelming emotions, you shut down. You go through the motions—present physically but absent emotionally. Your partner feels like they're living with a ghost. Intimacy (emotional and physical) evaporates.

What your partner experiences: Loneliness, rejection, confusion. "What did I do wrong? Why won't they talk to me?"

Irritability and Anger Outbursts

The chronic arousal of PTSD means you're always at a low simmer. Small frustrations—traffic, a messy kitchen, a comment from your spouse—ignite rage. You snap, yell, or say things you don't mean.

Afterward, you feel shame, which drives more withdrawal.

What your partner experiences: Fear, walking on eggshells, feeling unsafe. Children internalize the anger, believing it's their fault.

Hypervigilance and Control

You need to feel in control to feel safe. You dictate where the family sits in a restaurant (back to the wall, eyes on exits). You get anxious when your partner is late. You inspect the house for threats. This hypervigilance can feel suffocating to loved ones.

What your partner experiences: Frustration, feeling controlled, loss of autonomy. "I can't live my life without triggering your anxiety."

Avoidance of Intimacy and Vulnerability

Trauma teaches you that closeness equals danger. Being vulnerable with another person feels like handing them a weapon. So you keep your guard up, even with people who love you.

What your partner experiences: Loneliness, feeling shut out, wondering if you trust them at all.

Trust Issues and Jealousy

If your trauma involved betrayal (such as military sexual trauma, combat betrayal, or first responder misconduct), trust becomes nearly impossible. You might accuse your partner of lying or cheating without evidence. You check their phone, interrogate them about their whereabouts, assume the worst.

What your partner experiences: Hurt, defensiveness, resentment. Feeling like they're being punished for someone else's actions.

The Impact on Children

Children are especially vulnerable to the effects of a parent's PTSD.

They don't understand why Dad yells or why Mom won't hug them anymore.

They absorb the tension in the house and often blame themselves.

Research shows children of parents with PTSD are at higher risk for:

- Anxiety and depression
- Behavioral problems
- Difficulty regulating emotions
- Secondary traumatic stress (absorbing the parent's trauma responses)

Talking to Your Children About PTSD

Children do not need clinical explanations—they need honest, age-appropriate language that removes the most dangerous thing they will invent on their own: the belief that what is happening is their fault. A short, calm conversation, repeated as needed, does more to protect your child's emotional health than months of silence.

For young children (ages 4–8), keep it concrete and blame-free:

"Daddy has big feelings from his job that sometimes sneak up on him. It's never because of you, and it's never your job to fix it. You just have to keep being you."

"Mommy's brain learned to stay on high-alert to keep her safe. Sometimes it gets stuck that way. The doctors are helping her learn to turn it down."

For older children and teenagers (ages 9–17), they can handle more context:

"I have something called PTSD. It means my brain stores some memories differently because of things I saw in service. I'm in treatment for it. When I seem distant or get frustrated fast, that's the PTSD, not how I feel about you."

"If you ever feel scared or confused by how I'm acting, I want you to tell me or tell [trusted adult]. You don't have to carry that alone."

Regardless of age, repeat the three non-negotiables in every version of this conversation: it is not their fault, you are getting help, and they are safe to talk to you or another trusted adult about how they are feeling.

Resources for Children and Families

The following programs and materials are specifically designed for military and first responder families navigating a parent's PTSD:

• Sesame Street in Communities — "Talking to Children About War and Conflict" (sesamestreetincommunities.org): Free videos, tools, and conversation guides for parents of young children. Developed specifically for military families.

• Give an Hour — Family support and child counseling referrals for military and first responder families (giveanhour.org).

• Operation Purple — Summer camps and year-round programs for children of deployed and recently returned service members (nmfa.org/operation-purple).

• "My Dad Has PTSD" and "My Mom Has PTSD" — Children's books by Chad Crotty, written directly for the 6–12 age group.

• PTSD Family Coach App — The VA's free app includes a dedicated "Family Member" section with guidance on supporting children (mobile.va.gov/app/ptsd-family-coach).

• "Down Came the Rain" and "Brave Like Me" — Picture books for younger children about a parent's invisible wounds, recommended by military family advocates.

Communicating About Your PTSD

Open communication doesn't cure PTSD, but it prevents misunderstandings and reduces isolation.

Psychoeducation: Help Them Understand

Your loved ones need to understand that your symptoms aren't personal choices. You're not choosing to be distant or irritable—your brain is stuck in survival mode.

What to share:

- "I have PTSD. It's an injury to my stress response system. My brain is stuck in 'threat mode' even when I'm safe."
- "My symptoms include [specific symptoms they've witnessed]. These aren't about you or how I feel about you."
- "I'm in treatment. I'm working on this. But healing takes time."

Resources to share with loved ones:

- PTSD Family Coach app (U.S. Department of Veterans Affairs)
- Books: Loving Someone with PTSD by Aphrodite Matsakis; The Post-Traumatic Stress Disorder Sourcebook by Glenn Schiraldi
- National Alliance on Mental Illness (NAMI) family support groups

The Code System: Signaling Without Long Explanations

Create a simple system to communicate your state without lengthy explanations.

Example: Traffic Light System

Green: I'm okay. My nervous system is regulated. I can connect and be present.

Yellow: I'm on edge. I need space or grounding. Don't take it personally.

Red: I'm in crisis. I'm triggered or dissociating. I need you to

[specific action: give me space, hand me my grounding tools, check on me in 20 minutes].

Example conversation:

You: "Hey—I'm at Yellow. Need to step back for a bit."

Partner: "Got it. I'll be in the kitchen. Come find me when you're ready."

You: "Just 20 minutes. I'll come find you."

No long explanation needed. No guilt. Just honest communication.

"I" Statements vs. Blame

When discussing relationship issues, use "I" statements to avoid triggering defensiveness.

Instead of: "You never listen to me!" (blame)

Try: "Hey, it feels like I'm losing you when you're on your phone. Can we talk for a minute without screens?"

Instead of: "You're smothering me!" (blame)

Try: "I need a minute to breathe—it's not about you. Can we pick this back up in twenty?"

Timing Matters

Don't have big conversations when either of you is triggered, exhausted, or dysregulated.

Bad timing: Right after a PTSD trigger, late at night when you're both tired, during an argument

Good timing: When you're both calm, well-rested, and have privacy

Script example:

"I need to talk to you about something important. Can we set aside time this weekend when we're both rested?"

Setting Boundaries (For Both Partners)

Healthy boundaries protect both people in the relationship.

Boundaries for the Person with PTSD
You're allowed to:

- Take space when you're triggered (with communication)
- Say no to overwhelming situations (family gatherings, loud events)
- Decline to discuss trauma details if you're not ready
- Protect your recovery (limiting substances, maintaining sleep schedule)

Example scripts:

"I need to step outside for a few minutes. I'll be back."

"I'm not ready to talk about that deployment yet. I appreciate you respecting that."

"I know you want me to come to the party, but crowds are a trigger for me right now. Can we find a compromise?"

Boundaries for the Partner/Family Member

They're allowed to:

Have their own life, friendships, and activities

Express their feelings, including frustration or exhaustion

Not be your therapist or rescuer

Take care of their own mental health

Example scripts (for partners):

"I want to support you, but I need my own therapist to process what I'm going through."

"I understand you're struggling, but yelling at me isn't okay. I need you to take a timeout."

"I'm going out with friends tonight. I need that for my own well-being."

The Danger of Codependency

When PTSD dominates a relationship, codependency can develop. Your partner becomes hyper-focused on managing your symptoms, anticipating your triggers, walking on eggshells. They lose their own identity in the process.

Warning signs of codependency:

- Partner constantly monitors your mood
- Partner sacrifices their needs to avoid upsetting you
- Partner feels responsible for your recovery
- You rely on your partner to regulate your emotions

Solution: Both partners need independence, their own support systems, and their own lives outside the relationship.

Rebuilding Trust and Intimacy

If PTSD has damaged trust or intimacy, rebuilding takes time and intentional effort.

Start Small

Don't try to go from estrangement to full emotional intimacy overnight.

Rebuild in increments.

Examples:

- Week 1: Daily 10-minute check-in conversations
- Week 2: Holding hands while watching TV
- Week 3: Taking a short walk together
- Week 4: Sharing one thing you appreciated about each other

Physical Intimacy After Trauma

If trauma or PTSD has disrupted physical intimacy, go slowly and communicate constantly.

Strategies:

- Talk about sex outside the bedroom when you're not trying to initiate
- Discuss what feels safe vs. triggering (positions, touches, scenarios)
- Use explicit verbal consent: "Is this okay?" "Can I touch you here?"
- Establish a stop signal (verbal or physical) that either person canuse anytime
- Focus on non-sexual touch first: massage, cuddling, holding hands
- Consider sex therapy with a trauma-informed therapist

For survivors of sexual trauma:

Physical touch may be especially triggering. Your partner needs to understand that rejection of touch isn't rejection of them. Healing may require months or years of therapy before physical intimacy feels safe again.

Apologizing and Making Amends

If your PTSD symptoms have hurt your partner—outbursts, withdrawal, broken promises—you may need to make amends.

A genuine apology includes:

1. Acknowledgment: "I yelled at you last night. That was wrong."

2. Taking responsibility: "My PTSD doesn't excuse my behavior. I hurt you."

3. Expressing remorse: "I'm truly sorry."

4. Commitment to change: "I'm working with my therapist on managing my anger. I don't want to hurt you again."

5. Making amends: "What can I do to make this right?"

What not to do:

- Don't excuse: "I yelled because of my PTSD, so it's not my fault."
- Don't deflect: "Yeah, I yelled, but you provoked me."
- Don't demand forgiveness: "I apologized. You have to forgive me now."

Forgiveness takes time. Rebuilding trust takes consistent behavior change, not just words.

Understanding Secondary Traumatic Stress

Living with someone with PTSD can create secondary traumatic stress

(STS) in loved ones. They absorb your trauma symptoms. They become hypervigilant, anxious, or emotionally numb themselves.

Signs your partner/family may have STS:

Increased anxiety or hypervigilance

Nightmares or intrusive thoughts (sometimes about your trauma)

Avoidance of reminders of your trauma

Emotional exhaustion and burnout

Physical symptoms (headaches, insomnia, digestive issues)

What helps:

- Partners should seek their own therapy
- Partners need their own support groups (NAMI, PTSD family groups)
- Both partners practice self-care independently
- Professional help for both partners, not just the person with PTSD

What This Is NOT Asking of Your Partner

Asking your partner to understand your PTSD, absorb your symptoms, and stand by you through the hardest days of recovery is already an enormous request. But there is a line that support cannot cross, and it is important to name it plainly. Supporting you does not mean tolerating verbal abuse, physical intimidation, or coercive control. It does not mean erasing their own needs, abandoning their own mental health, or accepting chronic emotional neglect as a permanent condition. A partner can love you deeply, believe in your recovery fully, and still require that you treat them with basic dignity. These two things are not in conflict. In fact, the willingness to hold both—deep compassion for your struggle and clear boundaries around how you are treated—is what makes sustained partnership possible. If you find yourself justifying harmful behavior as a symptom, that is a signal to bring it directly into therapy.

Partner's Insight

"I used to think supporting him meant I had to absorb everything—the silence, the outbursts, the nights he wasn't really there. I didn't understand that I was disappearing in the process. The shift came when my own therapist helped me see that loving someone through PTSD and having boundaries are not opposites. They're the same act of respect. When I started naming what I needed—not as an ultimatum, but as a truth—something shifted in both of us. He began to take his treatment more seriously. And I began to feel like myself again. You cannot pour from an empty rucksack. That goes for partners too."—Composite account drawn from family support group experiences

When to Seek Couples or Family Therapy

Consider couples or family therapy if:

- Communication has completely broken down
- There's a pattern of escalating conflict
- One or both partners are considering separation
- Children are showing significant distress
- You've tried improving on your own without success
- Your individual therapist recommends it

Look for therapists trained in:

Cognitive-Behavioral Conjoint Therapy for PTSD (CBCT)

Emotionally Focused Therapy (EFT)

Gottman Method Couples Therapy (with trauma training)

What to expect in couples therapy:

- Learning communication skills
- Identifying negative patterns (pursue-withdraw, attack-defend)
- Processing how PTSD has affected the relationship

- Developing strategies to manage triggers as a team
- Rebuilding trust and intimacy gradually

If abuse is present: If there's physical violence, coercive control, or threats, individual therapy and safety planning come first. Couples therapy isn't safe or appropriate when abuse is occurring.

Relationships That Don't Survive

Not all relationships survive PTSD. Sometimes the damage is too deep.

Sometimes one or both people have changed too much. Sometimes the healthiest choice is to separate.

If you're considering separation or divorce:
For the person with PTSD:

This doesn't mean you're unlovable or broken beyond repair
Focus on your individual healing
Build a strong support network outside the relationship
Work with your therapist on grief and moving forward

For the partner:

Leaving doesn't make you a bad person
You've likely given everything you could
Prioritize your own mental health and safety
Seek support for yourself during this transition

If children are involved:

Tell children together in age-appropriate language
Reassure children it's not their fault
Maintain routines and stability for children

Continue co-parenting respectfully if possible
Both parents should be in therapy to process the separation
Building New Relationships When You Have PTSD
If you're single and have PTSD, dating feels daunting.

When you're ready to date:

You're in consistent treatment
You have healthy coping strategies
You're not looking for someone to "save" you
You can function independently

How to disclose PTSD:

Early dating: "I have some past trauma I'm working through in therapy. I might need space sometimes, and I have some triggers I'm managing."

Serious relationship: Share more specifics about your PTSD, treatment, triggers, and what support you need.

Red flags in potential partners:

- Someone who doesn't respect your boundaries
- Someone who tries to be your therapist
- Someone who treats you as fragile or broken
- Someone who gets angry when you're triggered
- Someone who pressures you to "get over it"

Practical Tools and Worksheets
Exercise 1: Relationship Inventory

Answer these questions:

1. How has PTSD affected my closest relationships?

2. What relationship patterns do I notice? (withdrawal, anger, control, etc.)

3. What do my loved ones need from me that I'm not giving?

4. What do I need from them?

5. What's one small step I can take this week to improve one relationship?

Exercise 2: Communication Card

Create a "What I Need When Triggered" card for your partner/family:

When I'm triggered:

- I might need: [space / physical comfort / grounding help / distraction]
- Please don't: [follow me / bombard me with questions / touch me /try to fix it]
- It helps when you: [give me 20 minutes alone / hand me my groundingtools / sit nearby quietly]
- I'll signal I'm okay by: [coming back to you / texting you / using our code word]

Exercise 3: Relationship Check-In Questions

Use these weekly with your partner:

1. On a scale of 1-10, how connected did you feel to me this week?
2. What's one thing I did this week that you appreciated?
3. What's one thing I could do differently next week?
4. Is there anything you need from me that you're not getting?
5. What's one thing you need for yourself this week?

Continuing the March

PTSD will test your relationships. It will push people away. It will make intimacy feel impossible. But relationships can survive PTSD—and even grow stronger—when both people commit to honest communication, mutual respect, and seeking help when needed.

Your partner who learns to recognize your triggers and doesn't take them personally.

Your child who learns that "Dad's having a hard day" doesn't mean "Dad doesn't love me."

Your friend who keeps texting even when you don't respond for weeks.

Your sibling who drives two hours to sit with you in silence.

These are the relationships that remind you that healing isn't a solo mission. That love can survive even the hardest battles. That you're worth fighting for.

Wayne's Insight

"My marriage almost didn't survive my PTSD. When you are going through something, it is almost like walking alone through a dark tunnel, and your vision narrows. You become consumed by your own pain. Blind to your partner's suffering.

Perhaps you share the same room and feel as though a wall separates the two of you. You on one side and your family and friends on the other side. But, here's the thing. They're exhausted. They feel alone raising their children, mostly by themselves. Maybe you were there, but physically there, but emotionally absent.

Then, one day, their silence became a roar. A shout of anger ultimately broke the self-absorption you held onto, which you equated with toughness, not by a chilling emptiness, signifying the quiet devastation of a spirit exhausted and a love that inattention had progressively worn away. The weight of a partner's unspoken burdens settled, heavy and suffocating.

The experience of couples therapy may inspire fear, yet it possesses the capacity to yield positive outcomes and provide valuable support. However, it's not a magic bullet, and its effectiveness relies heavily on both partners' willingness to be honest, vulnerable, and committed to the process, which can be incredibly challenging.

Chapter 10 End Notes & References

Monson, C. M., & Fredman, S. J. (2012). Cognitive-Behavioral Conjoint

Therapy for PTSD: Harnessing the Healing Power of Relationships.

Guilford Press.

Matsakis, A. (2014). Loving Someone with PTSD: A Practical Guide to Understanding and Connecting with Your Partner After Trauma. New

Harbinger Publications.

Gottman, J. M., & Gottman, J. S. (2018). The Science of Couples and Family Therapy: Behind the Scenes at the "Love Lab." W. W. Norton &

Company.

Sherman, M. D., Larsen, J., & Borden, L. M. (2015). "The Impact of PTSD on the Family." Professional Psychology: Research and Practice, 46(6), 419-425.

Figley, C. R., & Figley, K. R. (2009). "Stemming the Tide of Trauma

Systemically: The Role of Family Therapy." Australian and New Zealand

Journal of Family Therapy, 30(3), 173-183.

VA National Center for PTSD. (2022). "PTSD and Relationships." Retrieved from ptsd.va.gov/family/effect_relationships.asp

Nelson Goff, B. S., & Smith, D. B. (2005). "Systemic Traumatic Stress:

The Couple Adaptation to Traumatic Stress Model." Journal of Marital and Family Therapy, 31(2), 145-157.

Fredman, S. J., Vorstenbosch, V., Wagner, A. C., Macdonald, A., &

Monson, C. M. (2014). "Partner Accommodation in Post-traumatic Stress

Disorder: Initial Testing of the Significant Others' Responses to Trauma Scale (SORTS)." Journal of Anxiety Disorders, 28(4), 372-381.

PTSD Family Coach App. U.S. Department of Veterans Affairs. Available at: mobile.va.gov/app/ptsd-family-coach

PART IV

Advanced Terrain—Anger, Guilt, Substance Use, and Identity

The foundational skills are in place. The treatment work has begun. Part IV tackles the terrain that does not resolve on its own—the fire of chronic anger, the weight of guilt and moral injury, the pull of self-medication, and the fractured sense of identity that PTSD can leave behind. These chapters are demanding, but they address the issues that most often keep veterans and first responders from sustaining recovery. Move through them at your own pace, rucksack in hand.

11

Chapter 11: Managing Anger and Rage

Anger is one of the most misunderstood symptoms of PTSD. It's not just

"being mad." It's a white-hot rage that explodes over minor provocations. It's punching walls, screaming at people you love, road rage that puts you in danger. It's the shame afterward, the apologies, the promises to do better—and then doing it again.

If anger has become your default emotion, you're not weak or broken.

Your nervous system is stuck in fight mode, and anger is your brain's go-to response when it perceives threat (even when there isn't one).

This chapter will help you understand the neurobiology of PTSD-related anger and give you concrete tools to manage it.

Why PTSD Makes You Angry

The Survival Response Stuck on "Fight"

Remember the fight-flight-freeze-fawn response? When your brain perceives danger, it floods your body with adrenaline and cortisol, preparing you to fight or flee. In PTSD, your threat detection system

(the amygdala) is overactive. It sees threats everywhere. And for many people with PTSD, "fight" becomes the default response.

What's happening in your brain:

- Your amygdala (threat detector) is hyperactive, constantly scanning or danger
- Your prefrontal cortex (rational thinking, impulse control) is underactive
- Stress hormones keep you in a state of chronic arousal
- Your window of tolerance for stress is narrow—small stressors feel huge

Result: You go from zero to rage in seconds. A driver cuts you off, your kid leaves dishes in the sink, someone moves your stuff—and you explode.

Anger as a Shield

Anger is easier to feel than vulnerability. Underneath the rage, there's often fear, grief, shame, or helplessness. But those emotions feel too dangerous, too overwhelming. Anger feels powerful. It creates distance. It keeps people from getting too close and seeing how much you're hurting.

Ask yourself: What am I protecting by staying angry?

Anger as Injustice

If your trauma involved betrayal, moral injury, or injustice (military sexual trauma, wrongful punishment, being left behind by leadership, seeing rules applied unevenly), your anger may be rooted in righteous rage. You were wronged. The system failed you. People let you down.

That anger is valid. But if it's consuming your life and destroying your relationships, you need tools to process it without letting it control you.

The Cost of Unmanaged Anger

Health Consequences

Chronic anger damages your body:

- Increased risk of heart disease, high blood pressure, stroke
- Weakened immune system
- Chronic pain and inflammation
- Digestive issues
- Sleep disturbances

Relationship Destruction

Explosive anger destroys relationships. Partners leave. Friends disappear. Family members stop calling. Your kids learn to fear you or mimic your anger.

Legal and Financial Consequences
Anger can lead to:

- Assault charges
- Road rage incidents
- Getting fired from jobs
- Legal fees, fines, jail time

Self-Directed Anger

Sometimes the anger turns inward. You hate yourself for what you did or didn't do during your trauma. You punish yourself through self-harm, reckless behavior, or substance abuse.

The Anger Cycle (And How to Break It)

Understanding the anger cycle helps you interrupt it.

To break the cycle, you need to intervene at multiple points: catch the trigger early, manage the physical arousal, challenge the cognitive distortions, and develop alternative responses.

1. Trigger (external or internal—a sound, a memory, a feeling)
2. Physical arousal (heart rate spikes, muscles tense, adrenaline floods)
3. Cognitive distortion (catastrophic thinking, black-and-white thinking, jumping to conclusions)
4. Explosion (yelling, throwing things, physical aggression)
5. Aftermath (shame, guilt, apologies, promises to change)
6. Repeat

Figure Smart Diagram

To break the cycle, you need to intervene at multiple points: catch the trigger early, manage the physical arousal, challenge the cognitive distortions, and develop alternative responses.

Early Warning Signs: Catching Anger Before It Explodes

Most people think anger comes out of nowhere. It doesn't. There are physical warning signs before the explosion.

Physical warning signs:

- Increased heart rate
- Muscle tension (jaw, shoulders, fists)
- Rapid breathing
- Heat rising in your face or chest
- Restlessness, pacing

- Clenching fists or jaw
- Tunnel vision

Emotional warning signs:

- Irritability
- Feeling disrespected or dismissed
- Sense of injustice ("That's not fair!")
- Feeling cornered or trapped

Thought patterns:

Black-and-white thinking ("They always do this!" "Nobody respects

me!")

Mind reading ("They're doing this on purpose to piss me off!")

Catastrophizing ("This is going to ruin everything!")

Practice: For one week, track your anger. When you feel irritated or angry, note:

- What triggered it?
- What physical sensations did you notice?
- What thoughts went through your mind?
- What did you do?

Pattern recognition is the first step to change.

Cooling Strategies: Managing Anger in the Moment

When you notice early warning signs, use these strategies immediately:

The Timeout

When you feel anger rising, remove yourself from the situation.

How to do it:

- Tell the other person: "I'm getting angry. I need a timeout. I'll be back in 20 minutes."
- Leave the room, the house, the situation
- Do not drive (you're too activated)
- Do not drink alcohol (it lowers inhibitions)
- Do not ruminate on what made you angry (that keeps the fire burning)

Do this instead:

Walk (brisk physical movement burns off adrenaline)

Use 4-7-8 breathing (inhale 4 counts, hold 7, exhale 8)

Splash cold water on your face (activates the mammalian dive reflex, calming your nervous system)

Use a grounding technique (5-4-3-2-1 method from Chapter 4)

Return after 20 minutes. If you're still too activated, take more time.

Do not have important conversations while dysregulated.

Box Breathing

This slows your heart rate and activates your parasympathetic nervous system (the brake pedal for your stress response).

How to do it:

- Inhale for 4 counts
- Hold for 4 counts
- Exhale for 4 counts
- Hold for 4 counts
- Repeat for 2-3 minutes

Progressive Muscle Relaxation

When your muscles are tense (a common anger sign), deliberately tense and release them.

How to do it:

- Start with your fists: clench tightly for 5 seconds, then release
- Move to your arms, shoulders, jaw, legs—tense and release each muscle group
- Notice the difference between tension and relaxation
- The Ice Dive

This is a more intense intervention for severe anger.

How to do it:

- Fill a bowl with ice water
- Dunk your face in for 10-15 seconds (or hold an ice pack on your face)
- This activates the dive reflex, immediately lowering heart rate and blood pressure

Physical Exercise
Anger creates a surge of adrenaline. You need to burn it off.

Options:

- Go for a run
- Do push-ups, burpees, or jumping jacks
- Hit a punching bag (not walls, not people)
- Lift weights
- Intense yoga (not gentle/restorative—you need to burn energy)

Cognitive Strategies: Changing Angry Thinking
Your thoughts fuel your anger. Challenge the distortions.

Common Cognitive Distortions in Anger

1. Catastrophizing: "This is the worst thing ever!"

Challenge: "Is this really the worst? Or just frustrating? Will this matter in a week?"

2. Black-and-White Thinking: "They always disrespect me!" "Nobody listens!"

Challenge: "Is that true 100% of the time? Can I think of exceptions?"

3. Mind Reading: "They did that on purpose to piss me off!"

Challenge: "Do I actually know their intentions? Could there be another explanation?"

4. Should Statements: "They should know better!" "People shouldn't act like that!"

Challenge: "Says who? Is my 'should' a universal law or just my preference?"

The STOP Technique

When angry thoughts spiral, use STOP:

S: Stop. Pause. Don't react yet.

T: Take a breath. Inhale deeply, exhale slowly.

O: Observe. What's happening in my body? What am I thinking? What are the facts (vs. my interpretation)?

P: Proceed mindfully. What's the most helpful response right now?

Reframing: Finding Alternative Perspectives

Example 1:

Trigger: Your spouse left dishes in the sink.

Angry thought: "They're so disrespectful! They know this bothers me!

They don't care about me!"

Reframe: "They forgot. They're stressed about work. This isn't about me. I can calmly remind them or just do the dishes this time."

Example 2:

Trigger: Someone cuts you off in traffic.

Angry thought: "That asshole did that on purpose! I'll show him!"

Reframe: "They didn't even see me. Or maybe they're rushing to the hospital. It's not personal. Let it go."

Long-Term Anger Management Strategies

Managing anger isn't just about cooling down in the moment. It's about addressing the root causes and building a less reactive nervous system.

Therapy Specifically for Anger

Cognitive Processing Therapy (CPT) and Prolonged Exposure (PE) address the underlying trauma fueling the anger. (See Chapter 8.)

Anger Management Groups: Many VA hospitals and community mental health centers offer anger management groups specifically for veterans and first responders.

Cognitive Behavioral Therapy (CBT) for Anger: Focuses on identifying triggers, challenging distorted thoughts, and practicing alternative responses.

Medication

If your anger is severe and uncontrollable, medication may help stabilize your nervous system while you do the therapeutic work.

Options (discuss with a psychiatrist):

- SSRIs (sertraline, paroxetine) reduce irritability and impulsivity
- Prazosin (for nightmares and hyperarousal)
- Mood stabilizers (if anger includes manic or bipolar features)

Medication won't cure anger, but it can lower the baseline arousal so you have more capacity to use coping skills.

Lifestyle Changes to Lower Baseline Anger

Your nervous system's baseline state affects how easily you're triggered. If you're chronically stressed, sleep-deprived, or in pain, your anger threshold is lower.

Improve:

- Sleep (see Chapter 6): Aim for 7-8 hours. Poor sleep increases irritability.
- Exercise: Daily physical activity regulates mood and burns stress hormones.
- Nutrition: Limit caffeine (increases anxiety), limit alcohol (lowers impulse control), eat regular meals (low blood sugar = irritability).
- Limit triggers: If the news enrages you, stop watching. If certain people always trigger you, limit contact.

Mindfulness and Meditation

Mindfulness trains your brain to pause between stimulus and response. It strengthens your prefrontal cortex (impulse control) and calms your amygdala (threat detection).

Start with 5 minutes daily:

- Sit quietly
- Focus on your breath
- When your mind wanders (it will), gently bring it back
- Don't judge yourself

Apps: Headspace, Calm, Insight Timer
Repairing Relationships Damaged by Anger
If your anger has hurt people, you need to make amends.

Making It Right After an Outburst

After an outburst, making a genuine apology is not optional—it is the first step in rebuilding the trust your anger just damaged. As covered in depth in Chapter 10 ("Navigating Relationships"), a real apology moves through five elements: acknowledging exactly what you did, taking full responsibility without deflection, expressing genuine remorse, committing to change through concrete action such as therapy, and asking what you can do to make it right. What it never includes is an excuse. "I have PTSD" explains the biology behind the explosion—it does not transfer the responsibility for it. Rebuilding trust is not an event. It is a pattern of consistent behavior over time.

Rebuilding trust takes time and consistent behavior change.

When Anger Becomes Dangerous

If your anger includes violence or threats, you need immediate professional help.

Red flags:

- Physical violence toward people or animals
- Destruction of property
- Threats of violence
- Fantasies of revenge or violence
- Access to weapons while enraged

If you've been violent:

- Seek immediate help from a therapist or psychiatrist
- Consider voluntarily removing firearms from your home (ask a trusted friend to hold them)
- Join a domestic violence intervention program if appropriate
- Be honest with your treatment providers about the severity

If your partner/family is unsafe:

They need to prioritize their safety. Anger management is your responsibility, not theirs. They cannot fix you, and they should not stay in a dangerous situation hoping you'll change.

Practical Exercises

Exercise 1: Anger Log
For two weeks, track every time you feel irritated or angry.

Record:

- Date and time
- What happened (trigger)
- Physical sensations (heart racing, fists clenched, etc.)
- Thoughts ("They did this on purpose!")
- What you did
- Intensity (1-10 scale)

Look for patterns. What are your most common triggers? What time of day are you most reactive?

Exercise 2: Timeout Plan

Create a concrete plan for when you need a timeout.

My timeout plan:

- I'll say: [exact words you'll use]
- I'll go to: [specific safe place]
- I'll do: [specific calming activities—walk, breathe, cold water]
- I'll return after: [specific time—20 minutes minimum]

Share this plan with your partner/family so they know what to expect.

Exercise 3: Cognitive Challenging Worksheet

When you're angry, write down:
- **The situation:**
- **My automatic thought:**
- **Evidence for this thought:**
- **Evidence against this thought:**
- **Alternative explanation:**
- **More balanced thought:**

Example:

Situation: My spouse didn't text me back for 3 hours.

Automatic thought: They're ignoring me on purpose. They don't care.

Evidence for: They have their phone with them all the time.

Evidence against: They've been busy at work. They always respond eventually.

Alternative explanation: They got caught up in meetings.

Balanced thought: They're probably busy. I'll check in tonight instead of assuming the worst.

Exercise 4: Values Clarification

Ask yourself:

- What kind of person do I want to be?
- How do I want my kids to remember me?
- What do I value more than being "right" in an argument?

When anger surges, ask: "Is this reaction aligned with my values?"

Continuing the March

Anger doesn't have to control your life. With consistent work—therapy, medication if needed, daily coping skills—you can widen your window of tolerance and respond to triggers with less intensity.

You won't eliminate anger. That's not the goal. The goal is to feel anger without exploding. To notice it rising, pause, and choose your response. To repair relationships when you mess up. To become the person you want to be, not the person your trauma made you.

It's hard work. But you've done hard things before. You can do this too.

Wayne's Insight

"My anger almost got me killed. I was driving home from work one day, and some guy cut me off. Road rage took over. I chased him for miles, laying on the horn, flipping him off, screaming. He brake-checked me. I almost rear-ended him at 70 mph. When I finally got home, my hands were shaking. I realized: I could've died. I could've killed him. All over someone cutting me off in traffic.

"That was my wake-up call. I started working with a therapist on anger management. The first thing she had me do was track my anger for two weeks. I filled out a log every single time I felt irritated. The patterns were obvious: I was most reactive when I was sleep-deprived, when I skipped meals, and in situations where I felt disrespected. Just seeing the patterns gave me a sense of control—like, okay, this isn't random. There are triggers I can anticipate.

"I also learned that a lot of my anger was masking other emotions—fear, shame, grief. When my wife would ask me to open up about my deployments, I'd get angry because vulnerability felt too dangerous. Anger was easier. But in therapy, I learned to sit with those uncomfortable emotions instead of immediately converting them to rage.

"I'm not perfect. I still get irritable. I still raise my voice sometimes. But I haven't punched a wall. I haven't exploded at people. And when I do slip up,

I apologize genuinely and get back to using my tools. My anger doesn't run my life anymore. I do."

Chapter 11 End Notes & References

Chemtob, C. M., Novaco, R. W., Hamada, R. S., & Gross, D. M. (1997).

"Cognitive-Behavioral Treatment for Severe Anger in Post-traumatic

Stress Disorder." Journal of Consulting and Clinical Psychology, 65(1), 184-189.

Novaco, R. W., & Chemtob, C. M. (2015). "Violence Associated with Combat-Related Post-traumatic Stress Disorder: The Importance of Anger." Psychological Trauma: Theory, Research, Practice, and Policy, 7(5), 485-492.

Taft, C. T., Creech, S. K., & Murphy, C. M. (2017). "Anger and Aggression in PTSD." Current Opinion in Psychology, 14, 67-71.

Worthen, M., & Ahern, J. (2014). "The Association Between Childhood

Maltreatment and PTSD-Related Anger Symptoms Among Iraq and Afghanistan

Veterans." Journal of Traumatic Stress, 27(4), 477-481.

Siegel, D. J. (2010). The Mindful Therapist: A Clinician's Guide to Mindsight and Neural Integration. W. W. Norton & Company.

VA National Center for PTSD. (2022). "Anger and Trauma." Retrieved from ptsd.va.gov

McKay, M., Rogers, P. D., & McKay, J. (2003). When Anger Hurts: Quieting the Storm Within (2nd ed.). New Harbinger Publications.

Linehan, M. M. (2014). DBT Skills Training Manual (2nd ed.). Guilford

Press. (Emotion regulation and distress tolerance modules.)

12

Chapter 12: Guilt, Shame, and Moral Injury

Some wounds aren't visible. They're not in your body—they're in your soul. They're the memories that keep you awake at 3 a.m., replaying decisions you wish you could undo. They're the belief that you're fundamentally broken, unforgivable, unworthy of love or peace.

Guilt, shame, and moral injury are among the most painful aspects of PTSD. They're also the hardest to talk about because admitting them feels like confirming that you're the terrible person you fear you are.

But silence makes these wounds fester. This chapter will help you understand these emotions, distinguish between them, and begin the painful work of healing.

Understanding the Difference: Guilt vs. Shame vs. Moral Injury

Guilt

Guilt says: "I did something bad."

Guilt is about actions. It's remorse for a specific behavior—something you did or didn't do. Healthy guilt can motivate positive change. Excessive or irrational guilt becomes destructive.

Examples:

- "I should've checked the building one more time."
- "I shouldn't have followed that order."
- "I left them behind."

Shame

Shame says: "I am bad."

Shame is about identity. It's the belief that you are fundamentally flawed, broken, unworthy. Shame tells you that you don't deserve forgiveness, love, or peace. It's corrosive and isolating.

Examples:

"I'm a monster."

"I'm broken beyond repair."

"I don't deserve to be happy."

Moral Injury

Moral injury occurs when you do something—or witness something—that violates your core moral beliefs. It shatters your sense of right and wrong, your trust in authority, or your faith in humanity. Moral injury is common in combat, law enforcement, firefighting, and healthcare.

Examples:

- Following orders that resulted in civilian casualties
- Watching leadership make decisions that got people killed
- Being unable to save someone
- Witnessing atrocities and being powerless to stop them
- Discovering that the "mission" you believed in was based on lies

Moral injury often co-occurs with PTSD, but it's distinct. PTSD is about fear and survival. Moral injury is about betrayal, meaning, and conscience.

Where Guilt and Shame Come From in Trauma

Survivor's Guilt

You lived. Others didn't. Why you? What makes you deserving of survival when they died?

Examples:

- The soldier who survived an IED blast that killed their squad mates
- The firefighter who made it out of the building when their partner didn't
- The EMT who couldn't save a child

Survivor's guilt is irrational but powerful. Your brain tries to make sense of randomness by assigning blame—to you.

Actions Taken During Trauma

Sometimes guilt is about things you actually did:

- Killing in combat (even when justified)
- Following orders that harmed innocents
- Using force as a police officer or first responder
- Making split-second decisions that had tragic consequences

Your brain says: "I did that. I'm responsible. I'm a bad person."

Actions Not Taken

Sometimes guilt is about what you didn't do:

- Not saving someone
- Freezing instead of fighting
- Not speaking up against wrongdoing
- Surviving by hiding

Your brain says: "I should've done more. My inaction makes me complicit."

Betrayal by Leadership or Institutions

When leadership fails you—sending you into danger for no reason, covering up mistakes, punishing you for doing the right thing—it creates moral injury.

You believed in the mission, the institution, the oath. When that's betrayed, it shatters your worldview.

Shame About Your PTSD Symptoms

Shame isn't just about what happened during the trauma. It's also about how you've struggled since:

"Real warriors don't get PTSD."

"I'm weak for not being able to handle this."

"I've become a burden to my family."

The Neurobiology of Guilt and Shame

Why do guilt and shame persist even when rationally you know you did the best you could?

Your brain is stuck in a loop. The prefrontal cortex (responsible for rational thought) knows the truth: you were in an impossible situation, you made the best decision with the information you had, chance and chaos played a role. But the amygdala (emotional brain) doesn't care about logic. It's stuck on the emotional truth: something terrible happened, and you were there.

Rumination—replaying the event over and over—reinforces the neural pathways of guilt and shame. Every time you replay it, you re-traumatize yourself and strengthen the belief that you're to blame.

The Cost of Carrying Guilt and Shame

Depression and Suicidal Ideation

Shame is one of the strongest predictors of depression and suicidal thoughts. When you believe you're fundamentally bad and unworthy of love, life loses meaning. You may think: "The world would be better off without me."

Self-Punishment

You don't believe you deserve good things, so you sabotage yourself:

- Refusing to pursue happiness ("I don't deserve it")
- Avoiding close relationships ("If they really knew me, they'd leave")
- Engaging in risky or self-destructive behavior (substance abuse,reckless driving)
- Refusing treatment ("I don't deserve to feel better")

Isolation

Shame thrives in secrecy. You believe: "If people knew the truth about me, they'd reject me." So you hide. You withdraw. You carry the weight alone.

Relationship Damage

You push people away because you don't believe you're worthy of love.

Or you sabotage relationships to confirm your belief that you're unlovable.

Spiritual Crisis

If your faith was important to you, moral injury can destroy it. How can a loving God allow such suffering? How can you ever be forgiven? Some people lose their faith entirely. Others wrestle with it for years.

Challenging Irrational Guilt: Cognitive Reprocessing

Not all guilt is rational. Your brain may be blaming you for things outside your control.

Ask yourself these questions:

1. Did I have all the information at the time?

In retrospect, with all the information you have now, you can see other options. But at the time, in the chaos, with incomplete information, did you know what you know now?

Example: "I should've known there were civilians in that building."

Challenge: "Did I have intelligence saying there were? Or am I using hindsight to blame myself?"

2. Were there factors outside my control?

War is chaos. Emergencies are chaotic. You don't control other people's actions, equipment failures, or random chance.

Example: "If I'd gotten there faster, I could've saved them."

Challenge: "Was the delay my fault? Was traffic my fault? Was their injury survivable no matter what I did?"

3. What would I tell a fellow service member/first responder in the same situation?

We're often far more compassionate toward others than ourselves.

Example: "I froze. I should've fought."

Challenge: "If my buddy told me they froze during an ambush, would I call them a coward? Or would I understand that freeze is a normal trauma response?"

4. Am I holding myself to a superhuman standard?

You're human. You have limits. You can't save everyone, control everything, or predict the future.

Example: "I should've been able to save all of them."

Challenge: "Is it reasonable to expect one person to save multiple critically injured people simultaneously? Would I expect that of anyone else?"

Cognitive Processing Therapy (CPT) for Guilt and Shame

CPT (see Chapter 8) is particularly effective for guilt and shame. It helps you identify and challenge "stuck points"—beliefs that keep you trapped.

Common stuck points related to guilt and shame:

- "It was my fault."
- "I should have known."
- "I'm a terrible person."
- "I don't deserve to be happy."
- "I can't trust anyone."
- "The world is completely dangerous."

CPT teaches you to:

1. Identify the stuck point
2. Examine the evidence for and against it
3. Develop a more balanced, accurate belief

Example:

Stuck point: "It was my fault they died."

Evidence for: "I was in charge. I made the call to enter the building."

Evidence against: "I didn't plant the IED. I didn't know it was there. I followed protocol. Intel said the building was clear. Three other squad leaders reviewed the plan and agreed."

Balanced thought: "I made the best decision I could with the information available. The enemy planted the IED. Chance and chaos played a role. I'm not omniscient. Their deaths are a tragedy, but not my fault."

This doesn't make the pain disappear. But it loosens the grip of irrational guilt.

Moral Injury: When the Issue Isn't Irrational Guilt

Sometimes the guilt isn't irrational. You did something that violated your values—or you witnessed something that shattered your worldview.

This is moral injury, and it requires a different approach.

Moral injury isn't about changing your thinking. It's about making meaning, seeking forgiveness, and finding a way to live with what happened.

Acknowledging What Happened

The first step is facing it. Not minimizing, not rationalizing, not avoiding.

- "I killed someone." (Even if it was justified.)
- "I followed orders that resulted in innocent deaths."
- "I stood by while someone was harmed."
- "I was betrayed by people I trusted."

This is terrifying because it feels like confirming that you're a monster. But acknowledgment is necessary for healing.

Taking Responsibility (Without Drowning in Shame)

There's a difference between taking responsibility and self-flagellation.

Taking responsibility: "I made that choice. It had consequences. I have to live with that."

Self-flagellation: "I'm an evil person who deserves to suffer forever."

You can take responsibility for your actions while also acknowledging context: the circumstances, the pressure, the impossible choices, your state of mind at the time.

Seeking Forgiveness (From Yourself and Others)

Religious/Spiritual Forgiveness

If you have a faith tradition, seeking forgiveness through confession, penance, or spiritual practices can be powerful. Talk to a chaplain, priest, imam, rabbi, or spiritual leader.

Some people find that their faith is the only thing that offers peace.

Others find that their faith has been shattered by their experiences, and they have to rebuild or redefine it.

Making Amends

If possible, make amends:

- Apologize to someone you wronged (if it's safe and appropriate)
- Do volunteer work that aligns with your values
- Mentor others to prevent them from making the same mistakes
- Advocate for policy changes that address the systemic issues that contributed to your moral injury

Example: A veteran who carries guilt about civilian casualties volunteers with refugee organizations, helping the very population he once saw as the enemy.

Amends aren't about erasing what happened. They're about creating meaning from the pain.

Self-Forgiveness (The Hardest Part)

Self-forgiveness doesn't mean saying, "What I did was okay." It means saying, "I did something terrible. I carry that. But I'm more than the worst thing I've ever done. I deserve the chance to heal and become a better person."

Self-forgiveness is a process, not a one-time event. It requires:

- Acknowledging what happened
- Taking responsibility without self-destruction
- Committing to live differently going forward
- Practicing self-compassion (see below)

Self-Compassion: Treating Yourself as You Would a Struggling Friend

Self-compassion is the antidote to shame. It's not self-pity or letting yourself off the hook. It's treating yourself with the same kindness you'd offer a friend in pain.

Dr. Kristin Neff's three components of self-compassion:

1. Self-Kindness vs. Self-Judgment

Self-judgment: "I'm a monster. I'm irredeemable."

Self-kindness: "I'm struggling. I'm human. I made mistakes, and I deserve compassion as I try to heal."

2. Common Humanity vs. Isolation

Isolation: "I'm the only one who's done something this terrible."

Common humanity: "Many people have faced impossible choices. Many veterans carry guilt. I'm not alone in this."

3. Mindfulness vs. Over-Identification

Over-identification: "I am my guilt. It defines me completely."

Mindfulness: "Guilt is something I feel, not who I am. It's one part of my experience, not my entire identity."

Practical self-compassion exercise:

When you catch yourself in a shame spiral, pause. Put your hand over your heart. Say out loud:

- "This is really hard."
- "I'm not alone. Many people struggle with this."
- "May I be kind to myself in this moment."

It will feel awkward at first. Do it anyway.

When Professional Help Is Critical

Severe guilt, shame, and moral injury can lead to suicidal ideation. If you're thinking about suicide, get help immediately.

Call or text 988 (Suicide and Crisis Lifeline)

Text "HELLO" to 741741 (Crisis Text Line)

Call the Veterans Crisis Line: 988, then press 1

Therapies specifically for moral injury:

- Adaptive Disclosure (AD): Designed for moral injury in military populations
- Acceptance and Commitment Therapy (ACT): Focuses on values-based living despite pain
- Cognitive Processing Therapy (CPT): Addresses stuck points related to guilt and shame
- Impact of Killing (IOK) groups: Specifically for service members struggling with having killed

Writing and Ritual as Healing Tools

The Impact Statement

In CPT, you write an impact statement describing how the trauma affected your beliefs about yourself, others, and the world. Writing about guilt and shame in detail, then sharing it with a trusted therapist, can be incredibly freeing.

Letters You Never Send

Write a letter to:

- The person you couldn't save: "I'm sorry. I did everything I could."
- Yourself at the time of the trauma: "You were in an impossible situation. I forgive you."
- The person or institution that betrayed you: "You failed me. What you did was wrong."

You don't have to send these letters. The act of writing can be cathartic.

Rituals of Letting Go

Some people find healing through ritual:

- Writing down guilt on paper and burning it (symbolizing release)
- Creating a memorial for those lost
- Planting a tree in someone's memory
- Annual remembrance ceremonies

Rituals don't erase the past, but they can provide a sense of closure and honor.

Living with the Weight

Here's a hard truth: some guilt and shame may never fully go away. You may always carry it. But you can learn to carry it differently.

You can:

- Acknowledge it without being consumed by it
- Live a meaningful life despite it
- Use it as motivation to help others
- Accept that you're both imperfect and worthy of love

You can be someone who did something terrible and is also trying every day to be better. Both can be true.

Practical Exercises

Exercise 1: Stuck Point Challenge

Choose one guilt- or shame-related stuck point. Write:

- **My stuck point:**
- **Evidence for this thought:**
- **Evidence against this thought:**
- **Alternative explanation:**
- **More balanced thought:**

Example:

Stuck point: "I'm a monster for what I did."

Evidence for: "I killed someone."

Evidence against: "It was war. I was following lawful orders. They were armed and shooting at us. I've also saved lives. I'm kind to my family."

Alternative explanation: "I did something traumatic in a traumatic context. That doesn't define my entire character."

Balanced thought: "I carry the weight of having taken a life. That's heavy. But I'm not a monster. I'm a person who experienced war."

Exercise 2: Self-Compassion Letter

Write a letter to yourself as if you were writing to a dear friend who's struggling with the same guilt or shame.

What would you say to them? How would you offer compassion?

Then read it to yourself. Notice what emotions come up.

Exercise 3: Values Clarification

Identify your core values (honesty, loyalty, courage, compassion, service, etc.).

Ask:

- How did my actions during the trauma align or conflict with my values?
- How can I live according to my values now?
- What meaningful action can I take this week that reflects my values?

Living according to your values (even imperfectly) is the path forward.

Exercise 4: The Burden Stone
This is a symbolic exercise used in some moral injury programs.

- Find a small stone
- Hold it in your hand and think about the guilt or shame you carry
- Acknowledge the weight
- You can choose to carry it with you (keeping it in your pocket as a reminder that you carry this but it doesn't define you)
- Or you can choose a ritual to release it (throwing it into water, burying it, leaving it at a memorial)

Continuing the March

Guilt, shame, and moral injury are soul wounds. They don't heal quickly or easily. But healing is possible. You can learn to forgive yourself.

You can learn to live with what happened without being destroyed by it.

You can find meaning and purpose again.

You are more than the worst thing you've ever done. You are more than your trauma. You are someone who's survived unimaginable things and is still here, still trying. That takes courage.

Wayne's Insight

"The guilt almost killed me. I carried it for years—the weight of decisions I made in Bosnia, in Kosovo, in Haiti. I made calls that put people in danger. I followed orders that, looking back, I'm not sure were the right thing to do. I saw things I should've spoken up about but didn't because I was following the chain of command. For years, I believed I was a monster. I didn't deserve to sleep. I didn't deserve peace. I punished myself every single day.

"The turning point came in therapy when my therapist asked me: 'If your best friend came to you and told you he'd made the same decisions you made, in the same circumstances, what would you say to him?' I broke down. Be-

cause I'd never show my friend the cruelty I showed myself. I'd tell him he was in an impossible situation. I'd tell him he did the best he could. I'd tell him he was human, not a monster.

"That was the beginning of self-compassion. It didn't happen overnight. I still have days where the guilt is crushing. But I've learned to carry it differently. I've learned that I can hold two truths at once: what I did or didn't do was part of a terrible situation, and I'm also a person trying to do good in the world now.

"I volunteer with a veteran mentorship program now. I talk to younger vets about my experiences, including my mistakes and my regrets. I can't undo the past. But I can use it to help others. That's given me a sense of purpose again. The guilt is still there. But it's no longer the only thing I am."

Chapter 12 End Notes & References

Litz, B. T., Stein, N., Delaney, E., Lebowitz, L., Nash, W. P., Silva, C., & Maguen, S. (2009). "Moral Injury and Moral Repair in War Veterans: A Preliminary Model and Intervention Strategy." Clinical

Psychology Review, 29(8), 695-706.

Bryan, C. J., Bryan, A. O., Roberge, E., Leifker, F. R., & Rozek, D. C.

(2018). "Moral Injury, Post-traumatic Stress Disorder, and Suicidal Behavior Among National Guard Personnel." Psychological Trauma: Theory, Research, Practice, and Policy, 10(1), 36-45.

Maguen, S., & Litz, B. (2012). "Moral Injury in Veterans of War." PTSD

Research Quarterly, 23(1), 1-6.

Neff, K. D. (2011). Self-Compassion: The Proven Power of Being Kind to Yourself. William Morrow.

Resick, P. A., Monson, C. M., & Chard, K. M. (2016). Cognitive Processing Therapy for PTSD: A Comprehensive Manual. Guilford Press.

Gray, M. J., Schorr, Y., Nash, W., Lebowitz, L., Amidon, A., Lansing, A., ... & Litz, B. T. (2012). "Adaptive Disclosure: An Open Trial of a Novel Exposure-Based Intervention for Service Members with Combat-Related Psychological Stress Injuries." Behavior Therapy, 43(2), 407-415.

Shay, J. (2014). "Moral Injury." Psychoanalytic Psychology, 31(2), 182-191.

Tangney, J. P., & Dearing, R. L. (2002). Shame and Guilt. Guilford Press.

VA National Center for PTSD. (2022). "Moral Injury." Retrieved from ptsd.va.gov

13

Chapter 13: Substance Use and Self-Medication

The beer that helps you sleep. The whiskey that quiets the memories. The pills that numb the anxiety. The weed that takes the edge off. For many people with PTSD, substances become survival tools—ways to make it through another day, another night, another flashback.

But what starts as a coping mechanism becomes a new problem. Tolerance builds. You need more to get the same effect. Your life starts revolving around when you can drink or use. Relationships suffer. Work suffers.

Your PTSD gets worse, not better. And suddenly you're fighting two battles: PTSD and addiction.

This chapter addresses the relationship between PTSD and substance use, why it happens, and how to break the cycle without judgment or shame.

The Connection Between PTSD and Substance Use

The statistics are stark:

- 40-60% of people with PTSD also struggle with substance use disorder
- Veterans with PTSD are 2-3 times more likely to have alcohol use disorder
- Up to 30% of veterans seeking PTSD treatment also have substance use issues

Why is this connection so strong?

Self-Medication: The Brain's Desperate Solution

PTSD symptoms are overwhelming. Your nervous system is stuck in threat mode. You can't sleep. You have nightmares. You're hypervigilant, irritable, emotionally numb. Memories intrude at random times.

Substances offer temporary relief:

- Alcohol depresses your central nervous system, temporarily reducing hyperarousal
- Benzodiazepines (Xanax, Ativan) calm anxiety quickly
- Marijuana numbs emotions and physical pain
- Opioids provide escape from emotional and physical pain
- Stimulants (cocaine, meth) provide energy and focus when depression saps motivation

Your brain learns: "This substance makes me feel better (temporarily).

I need it to function."

Avoidance

Avoidance is a core PTSD symptom. You avoid places, people, and situations that remind you of trauma. You also avoid internal experiences—emotions, memories, physical sensations.

Substances are powerful avoidance tools. Drunk or high, you don't have to feel. You don't have to remember. You don't have to sit with the pain.

The problem: Avoidance prevents healing. Memories need to be processed, not buried.

Social and Cultural Factors

In military and first responder cultures, drinking is often normalized.

"Blowing off steam" after a tough deployment or shift. "Taking the edge off" with the team. It's bonding. It's expected. It's how you cope.

This makes it harder to recognize when drinking crosses the line from social to problematic.

How Substances Make PTSD Worse

In the short term, substances provide relief. In the long term, they make everything worse.

Disrupted Sleep

Alcohol might help you fall asleep, but it disrupts REM sleep (the restorative phase). You wake up groggy, unrested, more irritable. Your nightmares may actually increase.

Increased Depression

Alcohol and other depressants worsen depression over time. You feel worse when you're not drinking, so you drink more to feel better, creating a vicious cycle.

Impaired Judgment and Increased Risk-Taking

Substances lower inhibitions. You're more likely to engage in risky behavior: driving drunk, picking fights, saying things you regret, making impulsive decisions.

Interference with PTSD Treatment

Many PTSD therapies require you to be fully present, mentally and emotionally. If you're drunk or high, you can't do the work.

Substances block the emotional processing necessary for healing.

Some medications for PTSD (SSRIs, prazosin) interact dangerously with alcohol or other substances.

Tolerance and Dependence

Over time, your brain adapts to the substance. You need more to get the same effect. Eventually, you can't function without it. You experience withdrawal when you try to stop.

At this point, you're not using to feel good—you're using to avoid feeling terrible.

Warning Signs of Substance Use Disorder

Not everyone who drinks or uses substances has a disorder. But here are warning signs:

- Using more or for longer than intended ("I'll just have one drink" turns into finishing the bottle)
- Unsuccessful attempts to cut down or stop
- Spending a lot of time obtaining, using, or recovering from substances
- Cravings or strong urges to use
- Failing to fulfill obligations at work, home, or school due to use
- Continuing to use despite relationship problems caused by use

- Giving up activities you once enjoyed in favor of using
- Using in dangerous situations (driving, operating machinery)
- Continuing to use despite physical or psychological problems caused by use
- Tolerance (needing more to get the same effect)
- Withdrawal symptoms when not using

If you checked 2-3: Mild substance use disorder

If you checked 4-5: Moderate substance use disorder

If you checked 6+: Severe substance use disorder

The Trap of Shame

Shame keeps people trapped in addiction. You're ashamed that you "can't handle" PTSD without substances. You're ashamed that you've lost control. You're ashamed of things you've done while using. So you hide it. You lie. You isolate. And you keep using because that's the only way to numb the shame.

Breaking the cycle starts with dropping the shame. Addiction is a medical condition, not a moral failing. Your brain has been hijacked by substances and trauma. That's not weakness. That's neurobiology.

Breaking the Cycle: Strategies for Change

Acknowledging the Problem

You can't change what you don't acknowledge.

Ask yourself honestly:

Is my substance use helping or hurting my life?

Am I using to cope with PTSD symptoms?

Has my use increased over time?

Have I lied to people about how much I use?

Have I tried to cut back and couldn't?

If you answered yes to any of these, it's time to get help.

Integrated Treatment: Addressing PTSD and Substance Use Together

For a long time, the standard approach was: "Get sober first, then we'll treat your PTSD."

This doesn't work. If you stop using without addressing the PTSD that's driving the use, you'll relapse. The symptoms will be unbearable, and you'll reach for the substance again.

Current best practice: Integrated treatment that addresses both PTSD and substance use simultaneously.

Evidence-based integrated treatments:

Concurrent Treatment of PTSD and Substance Use Disorders Using

Prolonged Exposure (COPE)

Seeking Safety (focuses on safety and coping skills for both PTSD and addiction)

Integrated Cognitive Behavioral Therapy (combines CBT for PTSD and substance use)

These treatments teach you:

- How to manage PTSD symptoms without substances
- How to process trauma memories
- How to identify triggers and develop healthier coping strategies
- How to build a life worth staying sober for

Detox and Withdrawal Management

If you're physically dependent on alcohol or benzodiazepines, you cannot safely stop cold turkey. Withdrawal can be life-threatening (seizures, delirium tremens).

You need medical detox:

- Inpatient detox facility (hospital or specialized center)
- Medications to manage withdrawal symptoms (benzodiazepines for alcohol withdrawal, for example)
- Medical monitoring for safety

For opioids, medications like buprenorphine (Suboxone) or methadone can ease withdrawal and prevent relapse.

Don't try to detox alone. It's dangerous, and your chances of success are much lower without support.

Medication-Assisted Treatment (MAT)

For alcohol use disorder:

Naltrexone: Blocks the pleasurable effects of alcohol, reduces cravings

Acamprosate: Helps restore brain chemistry after quitting, reduces cravings

Disulfiram (Antabuse): Makes you violently ill if you drink

For opioid use disorder:

- Buprenorphine (Suboxone): Reduces cravings and withdrawal, blocks other opioids
- Methadone: Prevents withdrawal, reduces cravings
- Naltrexone (Vivitrol): Blocks opioid effects

MAT is not "replacing one drug with another." It's using medication to stabilize your brain so you can do the therapeutic work of recovery.

12-Step Programs and Peer Support

Alcoholics Anonymous (AA), Narcotics Anonymous (NA), and similar programs provide:

Community and accountability

Structure and routine

Peer support from people who understand

For some, 12-step programs are life-saving. For others, the spiritual component or emphasis on powerlessness doesn't resonate.

Alternatives to 12-step programs:

- SMART Recovery (science-based, focuses on self-empowerment)
- Refuge Recovery / Recovery Dharma (Buddhist-based)
- LifeRing Secular Recovery (secular, self-help)

Find what works for you. The best program is the one you'll actually attend.

Building a Sober Support System

You can't stay sober in isolation. You need people who support your recovery.

Who's in your sober support system?

Sponsor or mentor (from a recovery program)

Therapist or counselor

Sober friends (people who don't use)

Family members who support your recovery

Peer support groups

Who's not helpful?

- People you used with
- People who enable your use ("One drink won't hurt")
- People who pressure you to use
- Toxic relationships that trigger your PTSD

You may need to cut ties with people who sabotage your recovery. That's hard, but necessary.

Identifying Triggers and Building New Coping Skills

What triggers your urge to use?

Common triggers:

- PTSD symptoms (flashbacks, nightmares, hypervigilance)
- Stress (work, relationships, finances)
- Boredom

- Social situations (parties, gatherings)
- Emotional pain (grief, loneliness, anger)
- Environmental cues (driving past the bar, seeing old using buddies)

For each trigger, you need an alternative coping skill.

Example:

Trigger: Nightmares → Old response: Drink until I pass out → New response: Imagery rehearsal therapy, prazosin medication, grounding techniques

Trigger: Stress at work → Old response: Smoke weed after shift → New response: Call sponsor, go to the gym, practice deep breathing

Trigger: Hanging out with old friends → Old response: Drink with them →

New response: Suggest sober activities (coffee, hiking) or find new sober friends

Building a Meaningful Life in Recovery

Abstinence alone isn't recovery. Recovery is building a life you don't want to escape from. What gives your life meaning and purpose?

- Relationships with loved ones
- Work or volunteering
- Hobbies and interests
- Physical health (exercise, nutrition)
- Spiritual or philosophical growth
- Helping others in recovery

Addiction fills time. When you get sober, you have a lot of empty time.

You need to fill it with meaningful activities, not just white-knuckle through cravings.

Relapse Prevention

Relapse doesn't mean failure. It's a common part of the recovery process. But the goal is to learn from relapse and prevent it when possible.

Warning signs of relapse (before you actually use):

- Romanticizing past use ("It wasn't that bad")
- Isolation and withdrawing from support system
- Stopping therapy or meetings
- Increased stress without coping
- Complacency ("I've got this under control now")

If you notice warning signs, reach out immediately. Call your sponsor, therapist, or friend. Don't wait until you've used.

If you do relapse:

- Don't spiral into shame ("I'm a failure, I might as well keep using")
- Reach out for help immediately
- Get back into treatment
- Learn from it: What triggered the relapse? What can you do differently next time?

Recovery is not a straight line. It's messy. It's hard. But it's possible.

Special Considerations

Cannabis and PTSD

Marijuana is increasingly legal and often viewed as harmless. Some veterans swear by it for managing PTSD symptoms.

The research is mixed:

Short-term, cannabis may reduce anxiety and improve sleep

Long-term, regular use is associated with worse PTSD symptoms, dependence, and cognitive impairment

Cannabis can interfere with trauma processing (you need to feel emotions to heal them)

If you use cannabis for PTSD, talk honestly with your treatment provider. Be aware of the risks of dependence.

Prescription Medication Misuse

Not all substance use involves illegal drugs or alcohol. Prescription medications—opioids for pain, benzodiazepines for anxiety—can also be misused.

Signs of misuse:

- Taking more than prescribed
- Taking someone else's medication
- Using medication to get high, not just to manage symptoms
- Doctor shopping (getting prescriptions from multiple providers)

If you're misusing prescription meds, tell your doctor. There are safer alternatives.

When You're Ready to Quit but Your Partner/Friends Aren't

If your social circle revolves around drinking or using, getting sober means losing your community. That's terrifying.

You may need to:

- Find new sober friends (through recovery meetings, hobbies, volunteering)
- Set boundaries with old friends ("I'm not drinking anymore. If youcan't respect that, we can't hang out.")
- Accept that some relationships won't survive your recovery

It's painful, but your life depends on it.

Practical Exercises

Exercise 1: Substance Use Self-Assessment

Answer honestly:

- What substances do I use? How often?
- Why do I use? (To sleep? To numb emotions? To socialize?)
- Has my use increased over time?
- Have I tried to cut back? What happened?
- How is my use affecting my life? (Relationships, work, health, finances)
- Am I ready to change? If not, what's holding me back?

Exercise 2: Trigger and Coping Plan

Make a list of your top 5 triggers for substance use. For each, write:

• **Trigger:**

• **Old response (using):**

• **New coping skill:**

• **Person I can call for support:**

Example:

Trigger: Nightmares

Old response: Drink whiskey until I pass out

New coping skill: Imagery rehearsal therapy, call crisis line, practice grounding

Person to call: Sponsor (John), Crisis Line (988)

Exercise 3: Sober Activities List

List 10 activities you enjoy (or used to enjoy) that don't involve substances:

1. _______
2. _______
3. _______

When you have an urge to use, do one of these instead.

Exercise 4: Recovery Vision

Write a paragraph describing your life one year from now, sober:

- What does your day look like?
- Who are you spending time with?
- What are you proud of?
- How do you feel physically and emotionally?

This vision is your "why"—the reason you're doing the hard work of recovery.

The Path Forward

Recovery from both PTSD and substance use is one of the hardest things you'll ever do. There will be days you want to give up. Days you relapse. Days you feel like it's not worth it.

But thousands of veterans and first responders have walked this path and made it to the other side. You can too.

You deserve a life not controlled by substances. You deserve to feel your emotions without being destroyed by them. You deserve healing.

It starts with one day. One hour. One moment of choosing recovery over escape.

Wayne's Insight

Some people drink for years to manage their PTSD. Nightmares would resurface after each deployment, leading them to drink themselves to slumber. A six-pack a night could become a 12-pack. Then the drinking during the day—'just to take the edge off.' He told himself he had it under control. He wasn't some drunk sleeping under a bridge. He was a NCO with a successful career. But he was lying to himself.

"The breaking point came when his wife found him passed out in the garage at 2 p.m. on a Saturday. I'd missed my daughter's soccer game. She

looked at him and said, 'You're choosing alcohol over us.'He wanted to argue, but he couldn't. She was right.

He went to the VA and admitted. He had a problem. They enrolled him in an integrated PTSD and substance use program. For the first time, he was treating both issues at once. He learned that he was using alcohol to avoid my trauma, and that as long as he kept avoiding, I'd never heal.

But I have tools now. I have people I can call. And I have a life worth staying sober for. My relationship with my family is better than it's been in years. I sleep without whiskey. I'm present. I'm alive again, not just surviving."

Chapter 13 End Notes & References

Back, S. E., Foa, E. B., Killeen, T. K., Mills, K. L., Teesson, M., Cotton, B. D., ... & Brady, K. T. (2015). "Concurrent Treatment of PTSD and Substance Use Disorders Using Prolonged Exposure (COPE):

Therapist Guide." Oxford University Press.

Najavits, L. M. (2002). Seeking Safety: A Treatment Manual for PTSD and Substance Abuse. Guilford Press.

Norman, S. B., Trim, R., Haller, M., Davis, B. C., Myers, U. S., Colvonen, P. J., ... & Mayes, T. (2019). "Efficacy of Integrated

Exposure Therapy vs Integrated Coping Skills Therapy for Co-morbid

Post-traumatic Stress Disorder and Alcohol Use Disorder." JAMA Psychiatry, 76(8), 791-799.

Substance Abuse and Mental Health Services Administration (SAMHSA).

(2020). "PTSD and Substance Use Disorders." Treatment Improvement

Protocol (TIP) Series, No. 42.

McHugh, R. K., Hu, M. C., Campbell, A. N., Hilario, E. Y., Weiss, R. D., & Hien, D. A. (2014). "Changes in Sleep Disruption in the Treatment of Co-occurring Post-traumatic Stress Disorder and Substance Use

Disorders." Journal of Traumatic Stress, 27(1), 82-89.

VA National Center for PTSD. (2022). "PTSD and Substance Use." Retrieved from ptsd.va.gov

SMART Recovery. (2022). Retrieved from smartrecovery.org

National Institute on Drug Abuse (NIDA). (2021). "Treating Co-Occurring

PTSD and Substance Use Disorders." Retrieved from drugabuse.gov

14

Chapter 14: Employment, Purpose, and Rebuilding

Who are you when you take off the uniform? When you turn in your badge?

When you can't do the job that defined you for years?

For military service members, law enforcement officers, firefighters, and EMTs, work isn't just a job—it's an identity. It's who you are.

It gives you purpose, structure, camaraderie, and a sense of mission.

When PTSD forces you to leave that identity behind, or when you struggle to transition to civilian work, you face an identity crisis that compounds the trauma.

This chapter addresses the employment challenges specific to PTSD, the identity crisis that accompanies them, and how to rebuild a sense of purpose and self-worth beyond your traumatic career.

The Employment Crisis in PTSD

The statistics are sobering:

- Veterans with PTSD have higher unemployment rates than veterans without PTSD
- When employed, they change jobs more frequently and earn less
- Up to 44% of veterans report difficulty adjusting to civilian employment
- First responders with PTSD face similar challenges: difficulty holding jobs, conflicts with supervisors, termination

Why PTSD Makes Employment So Hard

PTSD Symptoms Interfere with Job Performance

Your symptoms don't disappear when you clock in. Hypervigilance: You're constantly scanning for threats, which makes it hard to focus on tasks. Open office plans, unexpected noises, people approaching from behind—all trigger your nervous system.

Concentration and Memory Problems: PTSD affects the hippocampus (memory) and prefrontal cortex (executive function). You forget instructions, miss deadlines, lose track of conversations.

Irritability: You snap at coworkers or customers. You have a short fuse with supervisors. You say things you regret.

Avoidance: You avoid meetings, crowded break rooms, team-building events. You isolate, which damages relationships with colleagues.

Sleep Deprivation: Nightmares and insomnia leave you exhausted. You can't think clearly. You make mistakes.

Difficulty with Authority: If your trauma involved betrayal by leadership, taking orders from a civilian boss may trigger intense reactions.

The "Civilian World" Doesn't Translate

The skills that made you exceptional in the military or first responder roles don't always translate to civilian jobs.

In the military, you led soldiers in combat. In the civilian world, that's described as "supervised a team." It sounds diminished.

In law enforcement, you made split-second life-or-death decisions. In a corporate job, people debate for weeks over PowerPoint slides.

The stakes feel too low. The work feels meaningless. You're bored, frustrated, and resentful.

Loss of Identity and Purpose

You were a Sergeant. A Firefighter. A Medic. That wasn't just your job—it was your entire sense of self.

Now you're... what? An insurance adjuster? A warehouse worker? A guy sitting in a cubicle doing spreadsheets?

You've lost:

- Your rank and the respect that came with it
- Your mission and sense of purpose
- Your tribe (the brothers and sisters in arms who understood you)
- Your identity (who are you if you're not a soldier, cop, or firefighter anymore?)

This identity crisis often hits harder than the PTSD symptoms themselves.

Stigma and Discrimination

Despite legal protections, PTSD-related stigma affects employment.

Some employers:

- View veterans or first responders with PTSD as "unstable" or "dangerous"

- Hesitate to hire someone with a mental health condition
- Terminate employees who disclose PTSD or need accommodations

You might face:

- Questions about your mental health in interviews (illegal, but it happens)
- Denial of promotions due to perceived "instability"
- Termination for behaviors related to unmanaged PTSD symptoms

The Americans with Disabilities Act (ADA) protects against discrimination, but enforcement is difficult.

Financial Stress Compounds PTSD

Unemployment or underemployment creates financial stress, which worsens

PTSD symptoms. You can't afford therapy, medication, or even basic needs. The stress triggers more symptoms, which makes job searching or job performance harder. It's a vicious cycle.

The Identity Crisis: Who Am I Without the Uniform?

Military and first responder identities are all-consuming. You're part of an elite group. You have a clear mission. You know your place in the hierarchy. You're proud of what you do.

Then you leave (voluntarily or involuntarily), and suddenly:

- You're just a civilian
- No one understands your background
- Your accomplishments feel invisible
- You don't know who you are anymore

Common thoughts:

- "I used to be someone. Now I'm nobody."
- "I saved lives. Now I file paperwork."
- "I'm useless in the civilian world."

This isn't self-pity. It's a real psychological crisis. Your sense of self was tied to a role you no longer have.

Rebuilding Identity: You're More Than Your Job

Identity work is hard. It requires letting go of who you were and discovering who you are becoming.

Step 1: Grieve the Loss

You lost something important—your career, your identity, your sense of purpose. You need to grieve that loss before you can move forward.

Allow yourself to feel:

Anger: "It's not fair that PTSD took this from me."

Sadness: "I miss who I was."

Fear: "What if I'm nobody now?"

Don't rush the grief. It's necessary.

Step 2: Separate Your Identity from Your Job

You are not just your job. You're a multifaceted human being with:

- Relationships (spouse, parent, friend, sibling)
- Values (honor, courage, compassion, integrity)
- Interests (hobbies, passions, curiosities)
- Strengths (leadership, problem-solving, resilience)

Exercise: List 10 things about yourself that have nothing to do with your military/first responder career.

Example:

1. I'm a father of two.

2. I love woodworking.

3. I'm loyal to my friends.

4. I have a dark sense of humor.

5. I'm good at fixing cars.

You are more than your trauma. You are more than your former job.

Step 3: Find New Purpose

Purpose doesn't have to come from paid employment. It can come from:

Volunteering (veteran service organizations, coaching youth sports,

animal rescue)

- Mentorship (helping younger veterans or first responders navigate their careers or PTSD)
- Advocacy (speaking out about PTSD, systemic issues, veteran rights)
- Creative pursuits (writing, art, music)
- Learning new skills (going back to school, learning a trade)

Ask yourself:

- What problems in the world bother me?
- How can I contribute to solving them?
- What would I do if money wasn't an issue?

Your purpose may evolve over time. That's okay.

Navigating the Job Search with PTSD

Job searching is stressful for anyone. With PTSD, it's exponentially harder. But there are strategies to make it manageable.

Translating Your Skills

Military and first responder skills translate to civilian jobs—you just need to reframe them.

Military → Civilian:

Led a squad of 12 soldiers → Managed a team of 12, responsible for training, performance evaluations, and mission success

Maintained and operated complex equipment → Technical proficiency in

[specific equipment], troubleshooting, preventive maintenance

Deployed to combat zones → Performed effectively in high-stress,high-stakes environments with limited resources

First Responder → Civilian:

Responded to emergency calls → Managed crisis situations, assessed risks, made rapid decisions under pressure

Provided emergency medical care → Delivered critical care in chaotic environments, maintained composure in life-threatening situations

Coordinated with multiple agencies → Collaborated with diverse teams, communicated effectively across organizations

Resources:

- Military OneSource (career counseling)
- American Corporate Partners (mentorship for veterans)
- Hire Heroes USA (resume help, job placement)

Disclosing PTSD: When and How You are not legally required to disclose PTSD to potential employers.

However, if you need accommodations, you'll need to disclose eventually.

When to disclose:

After you receive a job offer (you have more leverage)

If you need specific accommodations (flexible hours, quiet workspace, time off for therapy)

How to disclose:

Be matter-of-fact: "I have PTSD, which is a mental health condition resulting from my military service. I'm in treatment and manage it well. I may need [specific accommodation]."

Focus on what you bring to the table: "Despite this challenge, I have [skills, experience, strengths]. My PTSD has taught me resilience, adaptability, and the importance of mental health.

What not to say:

- "I'm broken."
- "I'm not sure if I can handle stress."
- "I might have flashbacks at work."

Frame PTSD as a manageable condition, not a disqualifying deficiency.

Requesting Reasonable Accommodations

Under the ADA, employers must provide reasonable accommodations for disabilities, including PTSD.

Examples of accommodations:

Flexible work schedule (to attend therapy)

Quiet or private workspace (to reduce sensory overload)

Modified break schedule (for grounding when triggered)

Noise-canceling headphones

Permission to position your desk facing the door

Modified uniform policy (if uniforms are a trigger)

To request accommodations:

- Notify HR or your supervisor in writing
- Provide medical documentation (from your doctor or therapist) confirming the diagnosis and need for accommodation
- Be specific about what you need

Employers cannot retaliate against you for requesting accommodations.

Managing PTSD Symptoms at Work

You can't eliminate PTSD symptoms overnight, but you can manage them so they don't derail your job.

Hypervigilance:

- Sit with your back to a wall, facing the door
- Use noise-canceling headphones
- Take walking breaks to discharge nervous energy

Concentration Issues:

- Use timers (Pomodoro technique: 25 minutes of focused work, 5-minute break)
- Write everything down (to-do lists, reminders)
- Limit multitasking; focus on one task at a time

Irritability:

- Take timeout breaks when you feel anger rising
- Practice deep breathing before responding to frustrating emails or colleagues
- Apologize genuinely if you snap at someone

Flashbacks/Triggers:

- Identify workplace triggers in advance (loud noises, certain smells,crowded spaces)
- Have a grounding plan (5-4-3-2-1 method, cold water, stepping outside)

- Communicate with a trusted colleague: "If I seem off, I might need a minute. I'll step away and come back."

Sleep Deprivation:

- Prioritize sleep hygiene (see Chapter 6)
- Talk to your doctor about medication for nightmares (prazosin)
- Use caffeine strategically (not after 2 p.m.)

When Your Job is the Trigger

Sometimes the job itself is triggering. Law enforcement officers with PTSD may be triggered by their own work. Veterans working in defense contracting may be triggered by military culture.

If your job consistently triggers you:

Talk to your therapist about coping strategies

Consider a job change (this isn't failure; it's self-care)

Explore disability benefits if you can't work

You don't have to stay in a job that's destroying your mental health.

Alternative Paths: When Traditional Employment Isn't Working

Not everyone with PTSD can succeed in traditional 9-to-5 employment, especially during active treatment. That's okay. There are alternatives.

Disability Benefits

If PTSD significantly impairs your ability to work, you may qualify for:

VA Disability Compensation (for veterans)

Social Security Disability Insurance (SSDI)

Workers' Compensation (if PTSD resulted from job-related trauma)

Applying for disability doesn't mean giving up. It means acknowledging that you need time to heal. Many people later return to work once their symptoms are better managed.

Self-Employment

Some people with PTSD thrive in self-employment:

- You control your environment, schedule, and workload
- You don't have to navigate office politics or authority hierarchies
- You can take breaks as needed without explaining to a boss

Options:

Freelancing (writing, graphic design, consulting)

Skilled trades (carpentry, plumbing, HVAC)

Small business ownership

Challenges:

Requires self-discipline and financial planning

Income may be inconsistent

No employer-provided benefits (you pay for your own healthcare)

Volunteer Work

If you can't work for pay, volunteering provides:

- Structure and routine
- Sense of purpose
- Social connection
- Resume-building

Options:

- Veteran service organizations (helping other vets)
- Animal shelters or therapy animal programs
- Youth mentorship or coaching
- Disaster relief organizations (Team Rubicon, The Mission Continues)

Going Back to School

Education can open new career paths and provide:

Time to heal while building skills

GI Bill benefits (for veterans)

Supportive campus veteran centers

A chance to start fresh in a new field

Practical Exercises

Exercise 1: Skills Inventory

List 10 skills you developed in the military or as a first responder.

For each, write how it translates to civilian jobs.

Example:

Military skill: Navigated complex logistics in resource-scarce environments

Civilian translation: Supply chain management, project coordination, problem-solving under pressure

Exercise 2: Values Clarification

Identify your top 5 values (e.g., service, loyalty, courage, family, integrity).

Ask:

How can I live these values in a civilian career?

What jobs or volunteer roles align with my values?

Exercise 3: Purpose Statement

Write a one-paragraph purpose statement:

"My purpose is to [what you want to contribute] by [how you'll do it] because [why it matters]."

Example:

"My purpose is to help veterans navigate PTSD by mentoring them through my own experience because no one should suffer alone."

Exercise 4: Job Accommodation Plan

If you're currently employed or job searching, write:

• **My biggest PTSD-related challenge at work:**

• **Accommodation that would help:**

• **How I'll request it:**

The Path Forward

Losing your military or first responder identity is painful. Struggling to find employment or purpose is demoralizing. But you are not defined by your trauma or your job. You have value beyond what you do for a living.

Your mission isn't over. It's just different now. Maybe it's raising your kids. Maybe it's mentoring other veterans. Maybe it's building furniture or writing poetry or simply getting through each day sober and present.

You get to define your purpose now. Not the military. Not the department. You.

That's terrifying and liberating at the same time.

Wayne's Insight

"When I retired from the Air Force, I didn't know who I was anymore.

For 23 years, I was Senior Master Sergeant Wayne Ince. I had rank. I had authority. I had a mission. Then I retired, and suddenly I was just...a civilian.

Wayne. Some guy trying to figure out civilian life. I applied for jobs, but I felt like a fraud. How do you explain 'led airmen in combat zones' on a resume when you're applying to be a mid-level manager at a company that sells widgets? It felt insulting.

"Eventually, I found work that aligned with my values: a government contractor that supports veterans. I wake up feeling like I'm contributing something meaningful. I've learned that my identity isn't tied to a uniform or a rank. It's tied to my values and how I show up for people. That's who I am now. A writer, An author, and a survivor."

Chapter 14 End Notes & References

Smith, M. W., Schnurr, P. P., & Rosenheck, R. A. (2005). "Employment

Outcomes and PTSD Symptom Severity." Mental Health Services Research, 7(2), 89-101.

Adler, A. B., Bliese, P. D., McGurk, D., Hoge, C. W., & Castro, C. A. (2009). "Battlemind Debriefing and Battlemind Training as Early

Interventions with Soldiers Returning from Iraq." Journal of Consulting and Clinical Psychology, 77(5), 928-940.

Sayer, N. A., Noorbaloochi, S., Frazier, P., Carlson, K., Gravely, A., &

Murdoch, M. (2010). "Reintegration Problems and Treatment Interests

Among Iraq and Afghanistan Combat Veterans Receiving VA Medical Care."

Psychiatric Services, 61(6), 589-597.

U.S. Equal Employment Opportunity Commission. (2022). "The ADA and PTSD." Retrieved from eeoc.gov

Kukla, M., McGuire, A. B., & Salyers, M. P. (2016). "Rural Veterans'

Vocational Needs and Experiences: A Qualitative Study." Journal of Rehabilitation, 82(4), 30-38.

Military OneSource. (2022). "Career Resources for Service Members."

Retrieved from militaryonesource.mil

Team Rubicon. (2022). "Veteran Employment and Purpose." Retrieved from teamrubiconusa.org

Hire Heroes USA. (2022). "Veteran Job Search Support." Retrieved from hireheroesusa.org

PART V

Crisis Management, Resources, and the Path to Growth

The earlier parts of this book have given you tools to understand, manage, and begin healing from PTSD. Part V shifts focus to three final, essential missions: knowing what to do when crisis strikes, navigating the systems and communities built to support your recovery, and understanding the remarkable possibility of post-traumatic growth. This is not the end of the march. For many veterans and first responders, it is where the march finally begins to feel like something worth taking.

15

Chapter 15: When Crisis Hits—Suicide Prevention

If you're reading this chapter because you're in crisis right now—because you're thinking about ending your life, because the pain feels unbearable, because you can't see a way forward—stop reading and call for help immediately.

Call or Text 988 (Suicide and Crisis Lifeline)

Veterans: Call 988, then press 1 (Veterans Crisis Line)

Text "HELLO" to 741741 (Crisis Text Line)

If you have a plan and means to act on it, go to your nearest emergency room or call 911.

This chapter exists because suicide is a real and present danger for people with PTSD. The statistics are grim:

- Veterans are 1.5 times more likely to die by suicide than non-veterans
- First responders face similarly elevated risks
- PTSD significantly increases suicide risk

But here's the other truth: Most people who survive suicide attempts are glad they survived. The crisis passes. The pain lessens. Life becomes bearable again. And then, eventually, good.

This chapter will help you recognize warning signs, develop a crisis plan, and understand what to do when you or someone you love is in immediate danger.

Understanding Suicidal Thoughts

Suicidal Ideation Is Common with PTSD

Having thoughts about suicide doesn't mean you're weak or crazy. It means you're in pain and your brain is desperately searching for a way to make it stop.

Types of suicidal thoughts:

Passive ideation: "I wish I would just go to sleep and not wake up." "I wish I'd died in that IED blast instead of coming home like this."

Active ideation: "I'm thinking about ways to kill myself." "I have a plan."

Passive ideation is concerning but not immediately dangerous. Active ideation with a plan and means is a psychiatric emergency.

Why PTSD Increases Suicide Risk

Emotional pain: The emotional pain of PTSD—the flashbacks, the nightmares, the guilt, the shame—becomes unbearable.

Hopelessness: You can't imagine ever feeling better. The future looks empty and dark.

Isolation: You've pushed everyone away. You believe no one cares.

Impulsivity: PTSD affects impulse control. A momentary spike in pain can lead to an impulsive suicide attempt.

Access to lethal means: Veterans and first responders often have firearms, which are the most lethal method of suicide.

Substance use: Alcohol and drugs lower inhibitions and increase impulsivity.

Moral injury and shame: The belief that you're fundamentally bad, unforgivable, a burden to everyone.

What Pushes Someone from Ideation to Action?

Research suggests three main factors:

1. Perceived burdensomeness: "I'm a burden to my family. They'd be better off without me."

2. Thwarted belongingness: "I don't belong anywhere. No one understands me. I'm completely alone."

3. Capability for suicide: Repeated exposure to danger and death (combat, first responder work) desensitizes you to your own death.

You're less afraid of dying.

When all three converge, the risk is highest.

Warning Signs of Suicide

Knowing the warning signs can save a life—yours or someone else's.

Immediate Warning Signs (Act Now)

Talking about wanting to die: "I can't do this anymore." "Everyone would be better off without me." "I wish I were dead."

Looking for ways to die: Researching methods, stockpiling pills, buying a gun, giving away possessions

Talking about feeling hopeless or having no reason to live

Talking about being a burden to others

Increasing substance use

Acting anxious or agitated: Restless, unable to sleep, pacing

Withdrawing from family and friends

Changing eating or sleeping patterns

Displaying rage or talking about seeking revenge

Taking risks that could lead to death: Reckless driving, walking into traffic, provoking fights

Saying goodbye: Visiting or calling people to say goodbye, writing a will, giving away prized possessions

Putting affairs in order: Making a will, buying life insurance, getting financial affairs in order

If someone shows these signs, do not leave them alone. Get help immediately.

Longer-Term Warning Signs (Require Attention)

Persistent depression

Talking about feeling trapped with no way out

Increased alcohol or drug use

Withdrawing from activities they used to enjoy

Dramatic mood swings

Previous suicide attempts

If You're in Crisis Right Now

If you're reading this and seriously considering suicide, I need you to do something for me: Delay.

Suicide is a permanent solution to a temporary problem. The pain you're feeling right now—as unbearable as it is—will not last forever. But you have to survive this moment to get to the other side.

Immediate Steps to Take

1. Call for help

988 (Suicide and Crisis Lifeline)

988, press 1 (Veterans Crisis Line)

Text "HELLO" to 741741 (Crisis Text Line)

Call a trusted friend, family member, therapist, or chaplain

Go to the nearest emergency room

2. Remove lethal means

If you have a plan, make it harder to act on:

Give your firearms to a trusted friend or family member (not just hiding them—actually removing them from your home)

Flush pills down the toilet

Give away medications that could be used for overdose

Remove ropes, belts, anything that could be used

3. Don't be alone

Call someone and ask them to come over

Go to a friend or family member's house

Go to a public place where you're around people

4. Use crisis coping skills

5-4-3-2-1 grounding (Chapter 4): Name 5 things you see, 4 you hear, 3 you can touch, 2 you smell, 1 you taste

Cold water: Splash your face with ice-cold water. Hold ice in your hands. Take a cold shower. (Activates the mammalian dive reflex, calming your nervous system)

Intense exercise: Do jumping jacks, run in place, do push-ups until you're physically exhausted. Burn off the adrenaline.

Breathe: 4-7-8 breathing (inhale 4 counts, hold 7, exhale 8). Repeat for 5 minutes.

Read your reasons to live list (see below)

5. Delay action for 24 hours

Make a deal with yourself: "I'll get through the next 24 hours. If I still feel this way tomorrow, I can reassess. But not tonight."

Most suicidal crises are time-limited. If you can get through the acute phase, the intensity often decreases.

Creating a Safety Plan

A safety plan is a written document you create when you're not in crisis to help you when you are. It's like a fire escape plan for your mental health.

Safety Plan Components:

Step 1: Warning Signs

List your personal warning signs that a crisis might be starting:

- I start isolating and not answering calls
- I start drinking more than usual
- I stop sleeping
- I have increased nightmares
- I start giving away my belongings

Step 2: Internal Coping Strategies (Things I Can Do Alone)

Go for a run

Take a cold shower

Listen to my grounding playlist

Use 5-4-3-2-1 method

Write in my journal

Watch a funny show (specific show: ________)

Step 3: People and Social Settings That Can Distract

Call my friend John (XXX-XXX-XXXX)

Go to the gym

Go to a coffee shop

Visit my sister

Attend a veteran support group meeting

Step 4: People I Can Ask for Help

List specific people with phone numbers:

Best friend: [Name], [Number]

Sibling: [Name], [Number]

Sponsor: [Name], [Number]

Therapist: [Name], [Number]

Chaplain: [Name], [Number]

Step 5: Professionals and Agencies I Can Contact

Therapist: [Name], [Number], [After-hours crisis number]

Psychiatrist: [Name], [Number]

Crisis Line: 988

Veterans Crisis Line: 988, press 1

Local crisis center: [Name], [Number]

Emergency room: [Nearest ER address]

Step 6: Making the Environment Safe

Firearms stored at [friend's name] house

Medications locked in safe, combination known only by [spouse/trusted person]

No alcohol in the house

Download a safety plan template: suicidesafetyplan.com or ask your therapist to help you create one.

Keep copies everywhere: on your phone, in your wallet, on your fridge.

Reasons to Live List

When you're in crisis, your brain can only see reasons to die. A "Reasons to Live" list, created when you're stable, reminds you why you're fighting.

Examples:

- My kids need me
- My dog depends on me
- I want to see my daughter graduate
- I promised my buddy I'd be at his wedding
- I haven't finished the book I'm reading
- I want to go fishing one more time
- Someone out there needs to hear my story to survive their own
- My pain might lessen if I give treatment more time

Write at least 10 reasons. Review it regularly. Add to it. Keep it with your safety plan.

If Someone You Love Is Suicidal

What to Do

1. Take it seriously

Never assume someone is "just talking" or "seeking attention."

Always take suicidal statements seriously.

2. Ask directly

"Are you thinking about killing yourself?"

This does not plant the idea. It opens the door for them to be honest.

3. Listen without judgment

Don't minimize: "You have so much to live for!" (They can't see that right now.)

Don't moralize: "Suicide is a sin!"

Don't dismiss: "You're just having a bad day."

Do listen: "I hear you. This sounds really painful. I'm here."

4. Don't promise to keep it secret

If they say, "Promise you won't tell anyone," you can't make that promise. Their life is more important than your promise.

Say: "I care about you too much to keep this secret. I need to help you get help."

5. Don't leave them alone

Stay with them until professional help arrives or until they're safe.

6. Remove lethal means

If they have access to firearms, medications, or other means, remove them. Don't just hide them—remove them from the environment.

7. Get professional help

Call 988 for guidance

Take them to the emergency room

Call their therapist or psychiatrist

If they refuse to go and you believe they're in immediate danger, call 911

8. Follow up

After the crisis passes, check in regularly. "How are you doing today?" "I'm thinking about you." "Want to grab coffee?"

Suicidal crises often recur. Your continued presence matters.

What NOT to Do

- Don't challenge them: "You won't really do it."
- Don't guilt them: "Think about your family!"
- Don't try to solve all their problems: "If you just did X, you'd feel better."
- Don't minimize: "Everyone feels like this sometimes."
- Don't leave them alone if they're in active crisis

Hospitalization: When and Why

If you're actively suicidal with a plan and means, you may need to be hospitalized. This isn't punishment. It's life-saving medical intervention.

Voluntary vs. Involuntary Hospitalization

Voluntary: You recognize you're unsafe and agree to go to the hospital for help.

Involuntary: If you refuse help but are actively suicidal, a family member, friend, or professional can petition for involuntary commitment

(often called a "5150" or "302," depending on the state). You'll be evaluated by a mental health professional. If you're deemed a danger to yourself, you can be held for 72 hours.

What Happens in a Psychiatric Hospital?

Assessment: A psychiatrist or psychologist evaluates your risk level.

Safety: Locked unit, no access to means of self-harm, 24/7 monitoring.

Medication management: If needed, medications are adjusted or started.

Therapy: Daily individual and group therapy focused on stabilization and safety planning.

Discharge planning: Before release, you'll create a safety plan and follow-up appointments.

Average stay: 3-7 days

Hospitalization isn't fun. But it's temporary. And it keeps you alive.

After a Suicide Attempt: Moving Forward

If you've attempted suicide and survived, you might feel a mix of emotions: relief, shame, anger, confusion.

Here's what you need to know:

You're not a failure for attempting. You were in unbearable pain and your brain saw death as the only escape. That's the PTSD talking, not reality.

You're not a failure for surviving. Most people who survive attempts report feeling glad they lived. You will too, eventually.

You need help. This isn't something you can power through alone.

Get into intensive treatment immediately: therapy, medication, support groups, possibly a partial hospitalization program (PHP) or intensive outpatient program (IOP).

Tell your treatment team everything. Don't minimize. They need to know how close you came so they can help you appropriately.

Rebuild your reasons to live. What kept you going before? What do you want to see or do? Create a new Reasons to Live list.

The Long Game: Building a Life Worth Living

Crisis intervention keeps you alive. But you also need to build a life worth living so you're not constantly in crisis.

This means:

Engaging in consistent trauma therapy (CPT, PE, EMDR—see Chapter 8)

Managing PTSD symptoms with medication if needed

Building meaningful relationships (Chapter 10)

Finding purpose (Chapter 14)

Developing healthy coping skills (throughout this book)

Connecting with peers who understand (support groups, veteran organizations)

You're not just surviving. You're working toward thriving.

Special Populations

Firearms and Veterans

75% of veteran suicides involve firearms. Firearms are the most lethal method—over 90% of firearm suicide attempts result in death, compared to less than 5% for overdose.

If you're suicidal and have firearms:

- Give them to a trusted friend or family member (not just locking them up—physically removing them from your home)
- Use a firearm storage program (some VA hospitals and police departments offer temporary storage)
- If you're unwilling to give them up entirely, at least separate guns from ammunition and give the ammunition to someone else

Your Second Amendment rights will still be there when you're stable.

But you need to be alive to exercise them.

Women, LGBTQ+ Veterans, and Minority Populations

Suicide risk isn't the same across all populations. Specific groups face additional challenges:

Women veterans: Higher rates of military sexual trauma, which increases suicide risk

LGBTQ+ veterans: Face stigma, discrimination, and higher rates of PTSD and suicide

Black and Hispanic veterans: Face systemic racism, lack of culturally competent care, and barriers to accessing VA services

If you're in one of these groups and struggling, seek out culturally competent providers and peer support specific to your identity.

Wayne's Insight

I haven't hurt myself on purpose, but I get how much you want to escape this pain. I swapped the good stuff for bad stuff. Things were pretty bad with my PTSD for a couple of years, and I felt stuck. Sleep was rough with those constant nightmares. I shut everyone out. Sleeping was the only reason I drank myself silly each night. I felt like I was too much for myself, my family, and everyone.

I was simply ready to give up.

Spirituality was the reason I couldn't. Faith's always mattered. I got a message and, instead of resisting my better judgment, I really paid attention. They jumped in at just the right moment, which was a lifesaver, and I really appreciate it.

"I called the Veterans Administration clinic. They talked me through it. They helped me create a safety plan. They convinced me to go to the Mental Health, where I was admitted to the psych evaluation. It was difficult. It was terrifying. But it saved my life.

"That was my rock bottom. And from there, I built my way back up. I got into intensive therapy. I connected with a peer support group of other veter-

ans who understood. I found a therapist who specialized in PTSD. I started taking medication. Slowly, very slowly, things got better.

"The bad thoughts still come sometimes, especially during low moments or when I'm triggered badly. But now I have tools. I have a safety plan. I have people I can call. I know the crisis will pass. And I have reasons to live—my family, my wife, the other veterans I mentor. I'm glad I'm still here. I almost wasn't.

But I am. And if you're reading this in crisis, I need you to stay too.

The world needs you. Your people need you. Fight through tonight. Call for help. You're worth saving. I have faith in you."

Chapter 15 End Notes & References

Bryan, C. J., & Rudd, M. D. (2018). "Nonlinear Change Processes During Psychotherapy Characterize Patients Who Have Made Multiple Suicide

Attempts." Suicide and Life-Threatening Behavior, 48(4), 386-400.

Joiner, T. (2005). Why People Die by Suicide. Harvard University Press.

Stanley, B., & Brown, G. K. (2012). "Safety Planning Intervention: A Brief Intervention to Mitigate Suicide Risk." Cognitive and Behavioral

Practice, 19(2), 256-264.

U.S. Department of Veterans Affairs. (2022). "Suicide Among Veterans and Other Americans, 2001—2019." Office of Mental Health and Suicide

Prevention.

Anestis, M. D., & Houtsma, C. (2018). "The Association Between Gun

Ownership and Statewide Overall Suicide Rates." Suicide and Life-Threatening Behavior, 48(2), 204-217.

988 Suicide and Crisis Lifeline. (2022). Retrieved from 988lifeline.org

Veterans Crisis Line. (2022). Retrieved from veteranscrisisline.net

Crisis Text Line. (2022). Text HELLO to 741741. Retrieved from crisistextline.org

Bryan, C. J., Mintz, J., Clemans, T. A., Leeson, B., Burch, T. S., Williams, S. R., ... & Rudd, M. D. (2017). "Effect of Crisis Response Planning vs. Contracts for Safety on Suicide Risk in U.S. Army Soldiers." Journal of Affective Disorders, 212, 64-72.

16

Chapter 16: Navigating the VA, Insurance Health

The bureaucracy of getting mental health care can feel like its own trauma. Endless paperwork. Long wait times. Confusing eligibility requirements. Insurance denials. The VA system that seems designed to frustrate you into giving up.

You've survived combat, emergencies, and trauma. Now you're facing a different battle: navigating healthcare systems that weren't built with PTSD in mind.

This chapter is your tactical guide to accessing care through the VA, private insurance, and community resources—including what to do when the system fails you.

Understanding the VA Healthcare System

For veterans, the VA is often the primary (or only) option for PTSD care. The VA has come a long way in PTSD treatment, but it's still a massive, often frustrating bureaucracy.

Am I Eligible for VA Healthcare?

Basic eligibility:

- You served in the active military, naval, or air service
- You were discharged under conditions other than dishonorable
- You meet minimum service requirements (varies by era)

You can apply even if you haven't received a VA disability rating yet. Priority Groups

The VA assigns veterans to priority groups (1-8) based on:

- Service-connected disabilities
- Income level
- Special eligibility factors (Purple Heart, former POW, Medal of

Honor, etc.)

Higher priority (Groups 1-4) = shorter wait times, lower or no co-pays

Lower priority (Groups 5-8) = longer wait times, may have copays

If you have a service-connected disability rating of 50% or higher, you're in a high-priority group.

How to Enroll

1. Apply online: va.gov/health-care/apply
2. Call: 1-877-222-VETS (8387)
3. Visit: Your local VA Medical Center
4. Mail: Print and mail VA Form 10-10EZ

You'll need:

- DD-214 (discharge papers)
- Social Security number
- Income information (for means testing)

Enrollment doesn't guarantee immediate access to care. You still need to schedule appointments.

Getting Your First PTSD Appointment

Once enrolled:

1. Schedule a Primary Care appointment

Your Primary Care provider can refer you to Mental Health. Some VA facilities allow direct scheduling to Mental Health, but many require a Primary Care referral first.

2. Request a Mental Health evaluation

At your Primary Care visit, say: "I need a referral to Mental Health for PTSD."

Be specific about your symptoms. Don't minimize. Don't tough it out.

The provider needs to know the severity.

3. Wait for your Mental Health appointment

Wait times vary by location. Some VA facilities can see you within days.

Others have months-long waits.

If the wait is too long, ask about:

Telehealth appointments (often shorter wait)

Community Care (see below)

Vet Centers (separate from VA hospitals, often shorter waits)

What to Expect at Your Mental Health Intake

Your first Mental Health appointment is an intake assessment. A clinician (psychologist, social worker, or psychiatrist) will:

Ask about your military service and trauma history

Screen for PTSD symptoms using standardized questionnaires (PCL-5,

etc.)

Assess suicide risk

Discuss treatment options

Create an initial treatment plan

Be honest. You're not impressing anyone by downplaying. They can only help if they know the full picture.

VA PTSD Treatment Options

The VA offers evidence-based treatments:
Cognitive Processing Therapy (CPT) (Chapter 8)
Prolonged Exposure (PE) (Chapter 8)
EMDR (Chapter 8)
Medications (SSRIs, prazosin, etc.)
Group therapy
Intensive PTSD programs (outpatient or residential, typically 2-8 weeks)

You have a right to request a specific therapy. If your provider isn't trained in it, ask for a referral to someone who is.

When the VA Wait Is Too Long: Community Care

If you can't get an appointment within 20 days (for mental health) or 28 days (for primary care), you may be eligible for Community Care

(formerly Choice Program).

Community Care allows you to see a private provider at VA expense.

How to access:

- Ask your VA provider to submit a Community Care referral
- Call the VA's Community Care program: 1-877-881-7618
- They'll help you find a provider in your area

Limitations:

- Provider must accept Community Care patients (not all do)
- VA pre-authorizes a certain number of visits
- You may still face wait times for non-VA providers

Vet Centers: A Hidden Gem
Vet Centers are separate from VA hospitals. They provide:

Free counseling for combat veterans and those with military sexual

trauma

No enrollment in VA healthcare required

No medical records (doesn't go into your VA file)

Shorter wait times

More informal, less institutional setting

Services:

Individual counseling

Group therapy

Family counseling

Readjustment counseling (for recent combat veterans)

Find your nearest Vet Center: vetcenter.va.gov

Vet Centers can't prescribe medication, but they can refer you to VA providers who can.

Filing a VA Disability Claim for PTSD

A VA disability rating provides:

- Monthly compensation
- Priority access to VA healthcare
- Potential for other benefits (vocational rehab, home loans, etc.)

How to File

1. Gather evidence:

Buddy statements (fellow service members who witnessed the traumatic

event or your symptoms)

Medical records (any documentation of PTSD symptoms during or after

service)

Personal statement (describe the traumatic event(s) and how PTSD affects your life)

2. File your claim:

Online: va.gov/disability

With a Veterans Service Officer (VSO): Free help from organizations

like DAV, VFW, American Legion

Mail: VA Form 21-526EZ

3. Attend the Compensation & Pension (C&P) exam:

The VA will schedule a medical exam with a VA examiner or contracted provider. They'll assess your PTSD symptoms and link them to your service.

Critical: Do not minimize your symptoms. Describe your worst days, not your best. The examiner needs to understand the full impact.

4. Wait for a decision:

Average wait: 3-6 months (sometimes longer)

5. Receive your rating:

PTSD is rated at 0%, 10%, 30%, 50%, 70%, or 100%

50% or higher: Considered "service-connected" with significant impairment

70% or 100%: Severe impairment, eligible for higher compensation and benefits

If Denied: Appeal

If your claim is denied or you receive a lower rating than expected:

You have one year to appeal

Work with a VSO to strengthen your appeal

Provide additional evidence (more buddy statements, medical records, personal statements)

Many claims are denied initially and approved on appeal. Don't give up.

Private Insurance and PTSD Care

If you don't qualify for VA care or prefer private providers, you'll need to navigate private insurance.

Understanding Your Mental Health Coverage

Under the Mental Health Parity and Addiction Equity Act, insurance must cover mental health at the same level as physical health. But there are still barriers.

Check your plan:

In-network vs. out-of-network providers: In-network = lower

copays. Out-of-network = higher costs, may not be covered.

Copays and deductibles: What you pay per session.

Session limits: Some plans cap mental health visits (often 20-30 sessions/year). Push back if you need more—parity laws require equal coverage.

Pre-authorization requirements: Some plans require approval before starting therapy.

Finding a Provider

1. Check your insurance company's provider directory (online or call member services)

2. Filter by specialty: Look for "PTSD," "trauma," "veterans"

3. Call providers: Verify they accept your insurance, have openings, and are trained in evidence-based PTSD treatment (CPT, PE, EMDR)

Red flags:

- "I use a general talk therapy approach" (not sufficient for PTSD)
- Not trained in trauma-specific therapies
- Doesn't understand military culture

What if No In-Network Providers Are Available?

If you can't find an in-network provider with PTSD expertise:

Request a "single case agreement": Ask your insurance to cover an out-of-network provider at in-network rates due to a lack of in-network options.

File a complaint: If your plan violates mental health parity laws, file a complaint with your state insurance commissioner.

When Insurance Denies Coverage

Denials happen. Common reasons:

"Not medically necessary"

"Exceeded session limits"

"Out-of-network provider"

How to appeal:

1. Request a written explanation of the denial

2. Gather supporting documentation: Letter from your provider explaining why treatment is necessary, clinical notes, research on treatment effectiveness

3. File an internal appeal (through your insurance company)

4. If denied again, file an external appeal (through an independent reviewer)

5. Contact your state insurance commissioner if the denial violates parity laws

VSOs and patient advocates can help with this process.

TRICARE (For Active Duty, Retired Military, and Dependents)

If you're active duty, retired military, or a dependent, you may have TRICARE.

TRICARE Mental Health Benefits:

No referral needed for mental health (you can self-refer)

Covers evidence-based PTSD treatments

Copays vary by plan (TRICARE Prime, Select, For Life)

Finding a provider:

Tricare provider directory: tricare.mil/find provider

Military OneSource: Free counseling (up to 12 sessions per issue, non-medical, confidential)

Active duty service members: PTSD treatment is free through military treatment facilities or TRICARE network providers.

Medicaid and Medicare

If you're low-income or disabled, you may qualify for Medicaid or Medicare.

Medicaid (low-income):

- Covers mental health services
- Benefits vary by state
- Many private therapists don't accept Medicaid due to low reimbursement rates
- Community mental health centers typically accept Medicaid

Medicare (65+ or disabled):

Covers 80% of outpatient mental health services (you pay 20% coinsurance)

No session limits

Most providers accept Medicare

Community Mental Health Centers

If you can't access VA care or afford private insurance:

Federally Qualified Health Centers (FQHCs): Sliding scale fees based on income

Community Mental Health Centers: Low-cost or free mental health services

University training clinics: Graduate students provide therapy under supervision, often at low cost

Find resources: samhsa.gov/find-help

Free or Low-Cost Resources

Give an Hour: Free mental health services for veterans and families (giveanhour.org)

Cohen Veterans Network: Free mental health care for veterans and families at Cohen Clinics (cohenveteransnetwork.org)

The Soldiers Project: Free therapy for veterans and families in select states (thesoldiersproject.org)

Wounded Warrior Project: Mental health services for injured veterans

(woundedwarriorproject.org)

When the System Fails You

Sometimes, despite your best efforts, you can't get the care you need.

Wait times are too long. Providers aren't available. Insurance denies coverage. The VA loses your paperwork.

What to do:

1. Escalate within the system

Patient Advocate (at VA facilities): File a complaint. They can sometimes expedite appointments or resolve issues.

VA Inspector General: For serious systemic problems (oig.va.gov)

Insurance ombudsman: File complaints about insurance denials

2. Contact your elected representatives

Your Congressional Representative or Senator can intervene on your behalf. VA facilities often respond faster when Congress is involved.

How to contact:

Find your representatives: house.gov/representatives and senate.gov

Call their local office

Explain the issue: "I'm a veteran with PTSD. I've been waiting X months for an appointment. I need help."

Congressional staff can submit inquiries to the VA on your behalf.

3. Use crisis resources

If you're in crisis and can't wait:

Call 988 (Suicide and Crisis Lifeline)

Veterans Crisis Line: 988, press 1

Go to the nearest ER

Walk into a Vet Center (they can see you same-day for crisis counseling)

4. Document everything

Keep copies of all paperwork

Track dates of appointments, referrals, denials

Save emails and letters

This documentation is crucial for appeals, complaints, and Congressional inquiries

5. Seek peer support while you wait

While navigating the system, connect with peer support:

Veteran support groups

Military family organizations

Online communities (r/Veterans, Rallypoint)

Peer support isn't a substitute for professional care, but it helps you survive the wait.

Practical Tips for Navigating the System

Be your own advocate

Don't assume the system will work. Follow up. Ask questions. Push back when necessary.

Bring a support person

Bring a trusted friend or family member to appointments. They can:

Take notes

Ask questions you forget to ask

Advocate for you if you're overwhelmed

Keep a symptom journal

Track your symptoms, triggers, and functioning. Bring it to appointments. It helps providers understand your needs.

Know your rights

- You have a right to see your medical records
- You have a right to request a different provider if the current one isn't helping
- You have a right to appeal insurance denials
- You have a right to file complaints about substandard care

Don't give up

The system is frustrating. But thousands of veterans and first responders successfully navigate it every year. You can too.

Wayne's Insight

"The VA system almost broke me before I even got into treatment. I enrolled in VA healthcare, but my first mental health appointment was three months out. Three months felt like an eternity, each second a heavy stone dragging him further into the abyss. My breath hitched, a cold sweat breaking out as the walls seemed to close in. My voice cracked with each desperate plea, the phone receiver growing slick in my sweaty palm. Nothing. A cold dread washed over me as each click and prompt seemed to steer me further into a labyrinth with no exit.

My breath hitched as I pushed open the familiar door, the sterile scent of antiseptic stinging my nostrils. I had no knowledge of Vet Administration.

A friend told me about the existence of Veteran assistant centers. They saw me fairly quickly and I walked in without a prior appointment. At the facility, a counselor assisted me in becoming stable and then referred me to an intensive PTSD program offered by the VA.

My first attempt to file a disability claim was unsuccessful. According to the examiner, my symptoms were not severe enough. My temper flared. However, I collaborated with a VSO, collected additional evidence such as buddy statements from my former comrades and letters from my doctors, and then filed an appeal. The VA granted my improved rating seven months later.

"Here's what I learned: the system is broken in a lot of ways, but there are people inside it who genuinely want to help. You have to be persistent. You have to advocate for yourself. And you have to know your rights. Don't let bureaucracy kill you. Fight for the care you've earned."

Chapter 16 End Notes & References

Chapter 16 End Notes & References

U.S. Department of Veterans Affairs. (2022). "Veterans Health Administration." Retrieved from va.gov/health

Veterans Benefits Administration. (2022). "How to File a VA Disability Claim." Retrieved from va.gov/disability

TRICARE. (2022). "Mental Health and Substance Use Disorder Care." Retrieved from tricare.mil/mentalhealth

Substance Abuse and Mental Health Services Administration (SAMHSA). (2022). "Find Treatment." Retrieved from samhsa.gov/find-help

Mental Health America. (2022). "Finding Help: Insurance and Cost Issues." Retrieved from mhanational.org

Cohen Veterans Network. (2022). Retrieved from cohenveteransnetwork.org

Give an Hour. (2022). Retrieved from giveanhour.org

National Alliance on Mental Illness (NAMI). (2022). "Navigating a Mental Health Crisis." Retrieved from nami.org

17

Chapter 17: Community Resources, Support Groups

Professional therapy is crucial. Medication helps. But recovery isn't just about clinical treatment. It's about connection, community, and finding your tribe—people who understand what you've been through because they've been there too.

This chapter is your resource guide: support groups, veteran service organizations, online communities, and practical tools to build your support network.

How to Find What You Need in This Chapter

This chapter covers a lot of ground. If you are in immediate crisis, go directly to the "Crisis Resources" table below—those numbers are available 24 hours a day, 7 days a week. If you are looking for peer support, scroll to "Peer Support Groups" and "Online Communities." For help with VA claims or legal matters, see "Veteran Service Organizations" and "Legal and Benefits Assistance." For family-specific resources, find "Family Support Resources." You do not have to read this

183

chapter straight through. Use it as a field manual—go to the section that fits your mission right now.

If you are in immediate crisis, use the table below. Do not read further. Make the call.

IMMEDIATE CRISIS RESOURCES
DO NOT WAIT — MAKE THE CALL

988 Suicide & Crisis Lifeline Anyone in crisis	**Call or text 988 • 24/7**
Veterans Crisis Line Veterans & service members	**Call 988, press 1 • Text 838255**
Crisis Text Line Anyone — text-based	**Text HELLO to 741741 • 24/7**
Safe Call Now First responders	**1-206-459-3020 • 24/7**
SAMHSA Helpline Substance use & mental health	**1-800-662-4357 • 24/7**
Military OneSource Service members & families	**1-800-342-9647 • 24/7**
National DV Hotline Domestic violence situations	**1-800-799-7233 • 24/7**

Save this page. Share it. It saves lives.

Figure 17.1 — Immediate Crisis Resources. Keep this page accessible. If you or someone you know is in crisis, make the call now — do not wait.

Resource	Who It's For	Contact
988 Suicide & Crisis Lifeline	Anyone in crisis	Call or text 988 (24/7)
Veterans Crisis Line	Veterans & service members	Call 988, press 1 • Text 838255 (24/7)
Crisis Text Line	Anyone (text-based)	Text HELLO to 741741 (24/7)

Safe Call Now	First responders	1-206-459-3020 (24/7)
SAMHSA Helpline	Substance use & mental health	1-800-662-4357 (24/7)
Military One-Source	Service members & families	1-800-342-9647 (24/7)
National DV Hot-line	Domestic violence situations	1-800-799-7233 (24/7)

Why Community Matters

PTSD thrives in isolation. When you're alone with your thoughts, the trauma narrative becomes louder, more convincing, more overwhelming.

Community disrupts that isolation. It reminds you:

- You're not alone
- Others have survived what you're going through
- Recovery is possible
- You're still part of something bigger than yourself

Research shows peer support improves PTSD outcomes, reduces suicide risk, and increases treatment engagement.

Types of Support You Need

You don't need just one type of support. You need multiple layers:
Clinical support: Therapist, psychiatrist, medical providers
Peer support: Other veterans or first responders with PTSD
Family support: Spouse, partner, parents, siblings
Spiritual support: Chaplain, faith community, spiritual practices

Practical support: Help with employment, housing, legal issues, benefits

Social support: Friends, hobbies, activities that bring joy

Think of your support network as a safety net. The more threads, the stronger it is.

Peer Support Groups

Peer support groups connect you with others who've experienced similar trauma.

VA-Facilitated Groups

Most VA medical centers offer PTSD support groups:

- General PTSD groups
- Combat-specific groups
- Military sexual trauma (MST) survivor groups
- Women veterans groups
- Anger management groups

Benefits:

Free

Facilitated by trained clinicians

Other members are veterans

How to find:

Ask your VA mental health provider for referrals

Call your local VA Medical Center and ask for the Mental Health department

Vet Center Groups

Vet Centers (separate from VA hospitals) offer:

Readjustment counseling groups for combat veterans

Bereavement groups

Trauma support groups

No enrollment in VA healthcare required

Find a Vet Center: vetcenter.va.gov

Veteran Service Organization (VSO) Groups
Many VSOs host local support groups:

- Disabled American Veterans (DAV)
- Veterans of Foreign Wars (VFW)
- American Legion
- Iraq and Afghanistan Veterans of America (IAVA)
- Wounded Warrior Project

These groups are peer-led (not clinician-led) and often more informal.

Online Support Communities

If in-person groups aren't accessible or you prefer anonymity, online communities provide connection.
Reddit:

- r/PTSD (over 100k members)
- r/Veterans (over 200k members)
- r/Military
- r/Military Sexual Trauma

RallyPoint: Social network for military members and veterans (rallypoint.com)

Team Rubicon Connect: Online community for Team Rubicon volunteers
(teamrubiconusa.org)

Private Facebook groups: Search "veteran PTSD support" or "first responder PTSD"
Benefits:
Anonymous
Available 24/7
Connect with people worldwide

Caution:

Not a substitute for professional help

Some groups have poor moderation (trolls, misinformation)

Crisis situations require real-time professional support (call 988)

12-Step and Recovery Groups (For Substance Use + PTSD)

If you're also navigating substance use:

Alcoholics Anonymous (AA) (aa.org)

Narcotics Anonymous (NA) (na.org)

SMART Recovery (secular, science-based) (smartrecovery.org)

Refuge Recovery / Recovery Dharma (Buddhist-based)

Many cities have veteran-specific AA/NA meetings.

Veteran Service Organizations (VSOs)

VSOs provide a range of services beyond support groups.

The complete Community Resource Directory—organized by category with websites and contact information for every organization in this chapter—is printed in **Appendix A** at the back of this book. It is formatted as a standalone reference designed to be scanned, photocopied, or shared. If you are helping someone else navigate PTSD recovery, hand them that page first.

COMMUNITY RESOURCE DIRECTORY

PEER SUPPORT

- **VA PTSD Support Groups**
  Free, clinician-led • va.gov

- **Vet Center Groups**
  No enrollment required • vetcenter.va.gov

- **Wounded Warrior Project**
  Peer support + wellness • woundedwarriorproject.org

- **Team RWB**
  Fitness + social connection • teamrwb.org

VETERAN SERVICE ORGS (VSOs)

- **Disabled American Veterans**
  Claims help, transport • dav.org

- **Veterans of Foreign Wars**
  Benefits, grants, community • vfw.org

- **American Legion**
  Advocacy + programs • legion.org

- **Iraq & Afghanistan Vets (IAVA)**
  Advocacy + mental health • iava.org

- **Team Rubicon**
  Mission-driven service • teamrubiconusa.org

- **The Mission Continues**
  Volunteer + leadership • missioncontinues.org

FIRST RESPONDER ORGS

- **Code Green Campaign**
  EMS mental health resources • codegreencampaign.org

- **Firefighter Behavioral Health**
  Peer support + prevention • ffbha.org

- **Badge of Life**
  Law enforcement support • badgeoflife.com

- **NAMI**
  Support groups + resources • nami.org

EMPLOYMENT & EDUCATION

- **Hire Heroes USA**
  Free job search + resume help • hireheroesusa.org

- **American Corporate Partners**
  Corporate mentorship • acp-usa.org

- **VA Vocational Rehab (VR&E)**
  Training + employment • va.gov

- **GI Bill**
  Education benefits • va.gov/education

FAMILY SUPPORT

- **PTSD Family Coach App**
  Free VA app for families • mobile.va.gov

- **Give an Hour**
  Free counseling for families • giveanhour.org

- **Blue Star Families**
  Community + programs • bluestarfam.org

- **Natl Military Family Assoc.**
  Resources + support • militaryfamily.org

SPECIALIZED SUPPORT

- **VA MST Coordinators**
  At every VA facility

- **Safe Helpline (DoD)**
  MST support • 1-877-995-5247

- **Women Veterans Call Center**
  1-855-829-6636

- **VA LGBTQ+ Coordinators**
  At every VA facility

- **OutServe-SLDN**
  Legal support • outserve-sldn.org

VA APPS (FREE)

COMMUNITY RESOURCE DIRECTORY

PEER SUPPORT

- **VA PTSD Support Groups**
  Free, clinician-led • va.gov
- **Vet Center Groups**
  No enrollment required • vetcenter.va.gov
- **Wounded Warrior Project**
  Peer support + wellness • woundedwarriorproject.org
- **Team RWB**
  Fitness + social connection • teamrwb.org

VETERAN SERVICE ORGS (VSOs)

- **Disabled American Veterans**
  Claims help, transport • dav.org
- **Veterans of Foreign Wars**
  Benefits, grants, community • vfw.org
- **American Legion**
  Advocacy + programs • legion.org
- **Iraq & Afghanistan Vets (IAVA)**
  Advocacy + mental health • iava.org
- **Team Rubicon**
  Mission-driven service • teamrubiconusa.org
- **The Mission Continues**
  Volunteer + leadership • missioncontinues.org

FIRST RESPONDER ORGS

- **Code Green Campaign**
  EMS mental health resources • codegreencampaign.org
- **Firefighter Behavioral Health**
  Peer support + prevention • ffbha.org
- **Badge of Life**
  Law enforcement support • badgeoflife.com
- **NAMI**
  Support groups + resources • nami.org

EMPLOYMENT & EDUCATION

- **Hire Heroes USA**
  Free job search + resume help • hireheroesusa.org
- **American Corporate Partners**
  Corporate mentorship • acp-usa.org
- **VA Vocational Rehab (VR&E)**
  Training + employment • va.gov
- **GI Bill**
  Education benefits • va.gov/education

FAMILY SUPPORT

- **PTSD Family Coach App**
  Free VA app for families • mobile.va.gov
- **Give an Hour**
  Free counseling for families • giveanhour.org
- **Blue Star Families**
  Community + programs • bluestarfam.org
- **Natl Military Family Assoc.**
  Resources + support • militaryfamily.org

SPECIALIZED SUPPORT

- **VA MST Coordinators**
  At every VA facility
- **Safe Helpline (DoD)**
  MST support • 1-877-995-5247
- **Women Veterans Call Center**
  1-855-829-6636
- **VA LGBTQ+ Coordinators**
  At every VA facility
- **OutServe-SLDN**
  Legal support • outserve-sldn.org

VA APPS (FREE)

Figure 17.2 — Community Resource Directory. All organizations listed are free or low-cost. No referral is required to call any of these numbers.

Major VSOs

Disabled American Veterans (DAV)

Free help filing VA disability claims

Transportation to VA appointments

Local chapters nationwide

Website: dav.org

Veterans of Foreign Wars (VFW)

VA claims assistance

Financial grants for veterans in need

Local posts with social events

Website: vfw.org

American Legion

VA benefits assistance

Veteran advocacy

Community programs

Website: legion.org

Wounded Warrior Project (WWP)

Mental health programs

Peer support

Long-term rehabilitation services

Financial assistance

Website: woundedwarriorproject.org

Iraq and Afghanistan Veterans of America (IAVA)

Advocacy for recent veterans

Community events

Mental health resources

Website: iava.org

Team Rubicon

Disaster relief volunteer organization

Provides purpose and mission for veterans

Strong peer community

Website: teamrubiconusa.org

The Mission Continues

Volunteer service opportunities

Leadership development

Community platoons (local service teams)

Website: missioncontinues.org

Team Red, White & Blue (Team RWB)

Physical fitness and social connection

Local chapters with group workouts and events

Website: teamrwb.org

Service-Specific Organizations

Air Force: Air Force Sergeants Association (hqafsa.org)

Army: Association of the United States Army (ausa.org)

Navy: Navy-Marine Corps Relief Society (nmcrs.org)

Marine Corps: Marine Corps League (mcleague.org)

Coast Guard: Coast Guard Foundation (coastguardfoundation.org)

First Responder Organizations

National Alliance on Mental Illness (NAMI): Support groups and resources for first responders (nami.org)

Code Green Campaign: Mental health resources for EMS and first responders (codegreencampaign.org)

Firefighter Behavioral Health Alliance: Peer support and suicide prevention (ffbha.org)

Badge of Life: Mental health support for law enforcement (badgeoflife.com)

Safe Call Now: 24/7 crisis line for first responders: 1-206-459-3020 (safecallnow.org)

Crisis Resources (Immediate Help)

988 Suicide and Crisis Lifeline: Call or text 988 (24/7)

Veterans Crisis Line: Call 988, press 1 / Text 838255 / Chat at veteranscrisisline.net (24/7)

Crisis Text Line: Text HELLO to 741741 (24/7)

SAMHSA National Helpline (substance use and mental health):

1-800-662-4357 (24/7)

Military OneSource: 1-800-342-9647 (non-medical counseling, 24/7 support)

Safe Call Now (first responders): 1-206-459-3020

National Domestic Violence Hotline: 1-800-799-7233 (if your PTSD symptoms include violence at home)

Legal and Benefits Assistance

Veteran Legal Services:
Many law schools offer free legal clinics for veterans (housing issues, family law, benefits appeals, discharge upgrades).
Find a clinic: americanbar.org/veterans
VA Regional Offices:
Help with benefits questions, disability claims, education benefits (GI
Bill), home loans.

Find your regional office: va.gov/find-locations

Homeless Veteran Services:
If you're homeless or at risk:
VA Homeless Programs: 1-877-424-3838 or va.gov/homeless
HUD-VASH (Housing and Urban Development-VA Supportive Housing): Vouchers for permanent housing + case management
Stand Downs: Community events offering services, supplies, and referrals to homeless veterans

Employment and Education Resources

Hire Heroes USA: Free job search assistance, resume help, interview coaching (hireheroesusa.org)

American Corporate Partners (ACP): One-on-one mentorship with corporate professionals (acp-usa.org)

Military OneSource: Career counseling, resume building, job search support (militaryonesource.mil)

VA Vocational Rehabilitation (VR&E): Education, training, employment support for veterans with service-connected disabilities

(va.gov/careers-employment/vocational-rehabilitation)

GI Bill: Education benefits for veterans (va.gov/education)

Family Support Resources

PTSD Family Coach App: Free VA app with information and tools for families of those with PTSD (mobile.va.gov/app/ptsd-family-coach)

National Military Family Association: Support and resources for military families (militaryfamily.org)

Give an Hour: Free counseling for military families (giveanhour.org)

Blue Star Families: Community programs and support for military families (bluestarfam.org)

Military Family Advisory Network: Resources and support for military families (militaryfamilyadvisorynetwork.org)

Financial Assistance

If you're struggling financially due to PTSD or unemployment:

Army Emergency Relief (AER): Financial assistance for active duty Army, retirees, and families (armyemergencyrelief.org)

Navy-Marine Corps Relief Society: Interest-free loans and grants (nmcrs.org)

Air Force Aid Society: Financial assistance for Air Force members and families (afas.org)

Coast Guard Mutual Assistance: Financial assistance for Coast Guard families (cgmahq.org)

Veterans of Foreign Wars (VFW): Emergency financial assistance program (vfw.org/assistance)

Modest Needs: Short-term financial assistance for working families (modestneeds.org)

Specialized Support

Military Sexual Trauma (MST) Support:

- VA MST Coordinators at every VA facility
- Vet Center MST counseling
- Safe Helpline (Department of Defense): 1-877-995-5247 or safehelpline.org

Women Veterans:

VA Women Veterans Program Managers at every facility
Women Veterans Call Center: 1-855-829-6636
Service Women's Action Network (SWAN): servicewomen.org

LGBTQ+ Veterans:

- VA LGBTQ+ Veteran Care Coordinator at every facility
- OutServe-SLDN (legal support): outserve-sldn.org
- Modern Military Association of America: modernmilitary.org

Minority Veterans:

- VA Minority Veterans Program Coordinators
- Culturally-specific VSO chapters (e.g., Montford Point Marine
- Association for Black Marines, American GI Forum for Hispanic veterans)
- Books, Apps, and Self-Help Resources

Books:
The Body Keeps the Score by Bessel van der Kolk
Achilles in Vietnam by Jonathan Shay
Waking the Tiger by Peter Levine
The PTSD Workbook by Mary Beth Williams
Warrior's Journey Home by Bret Moore
Apps (many are free):

PTSD Coach (VA): Self-help for PTSD symptoms

Mindfulness Coach (VA): Meditation and mindfulness training

PE Coach (VA): Companion app for Prolonged Exposure therapy

CPT Coach (VA): Companion app for Cognitive Processing Therapy

Insomnia Coach (VA): Sleep improvement tools

Calm / Headspace: Meditation and relaxation

Download VA apps: mobile.va.gov
Online Courses:
PTSD: National Center for PTSD: Free self-paced courses (ptsd.va.gov)
Make the Connection: Veteran stories and resources (maketheconnection.net)
Building Your Personal Support Team
You need a team. Here's how to build it:
Step 1: Identify your needs
What support do you need right now?

- Clinical (therapy, medication)
- Peer (veteran buddies who understand)
- Practical (help with VA claims, employment)
- Social (people to do non-trauma-related activities with)
- Spiritual (chaplain, faith community)

Step 2: Reach out
Choose one resource from this chapter and make contact this week:

- Join one support group
- Call one VSO
- Download one VA app
- Attend one Team RWB workout

Step 3: Show up consistently
Support networks are built over time. Go to the group. Answer the texts.
Show up even when you don't feel like it.
Step 4: Give back
As you heal, help others. Mentor a newer veteran. Share your story.

Volunteer. Giving back creates purpose and solidifies your own recovery.

Overcoming Barriers to Seeking Support

"I don't want to burden anyone."

→ People in these communities want to help. That's why they're there.

You're not a burden—you're the reason they exist.

"I'm too messed up."

→ No one is "too messed up" for support. These groups exist specifically for people who are struggling.

"I tried a group once and didn't like it."

→ Not every group is a good fit. Try a different one. It might take 2-3 tries to find your people.

"I don't have time."

→ One hour a week. That's all most groups require. You have time—you're choosing to prioritize other things. Prioritize your recovery.

"Virtual groups aren't the same as in-person."

→ True, but virtual is better than nothing. Start there if in-person isn't accessible.

Final Thoughts: Your Tribe is Out There

You're not the first person to walk this path. Thousands of veterans and first responders have navigated PTSD recovery before you. They're out there, waiting to welcome you into the tribe.

But you have to take the first step. Pick up the phone. Send the email.

Show up to the meeting. Walk through the door.

Your people are waiting.

Wayne's Insight

"I thought I could handle it alone. I thought admitting I needed help meant I was weak. But isolation was killing me. I was drinking alone, avoiding friends, pushing my family away. I was convinced no one could understand what I was going through.

"If you're reading this and you're isolated, I'm telling you: reach out. Find your people. They're out there. You don't have to do this alone. You weren't meant to."

Chapter 17 End Notes & References

Berke, D. S., Kline, N. K., Wachen, J. S., McLean, C. P., Yarvis, J. S., Mintz, J., ... & Foa, E. B. (2019). "Predictors of Attendance and Dropout in Three Randomized Controlled Trials of PTSD Treatment for Active Duty Service Members." Behaviour Research and Therapy, 118, 7-17.

Pfeiffer, P. N., Heisler, M., Piette, J. D., Rogers, M. A., & Valenstein, M. (2011). "Efficacy of Peer Support Interventions for Depression: A Meta-Analysis." General Hospital Psychiatry, 33(1), 29-36.

VA National Center for PTSD. (2022). "Resources for Veterans." Retrieved from ptsd.va.gov

Team Rubicon. (2022). Retrieved from teamrubiconusa.org

The Mission Continues. (2022). Retrieved from missioncontinues.org

Veterans of Foreign Wars (VFW). (2022). Retrieved from vfw.org

Disabled American Veterans (DAV). (2022). Retrieved from dav.org

988 Suicide and Crisis Lifeline. (2022). Retrieved from 988lifeline.org

Military OneSource. (2022). Retrieved from militaryonesource.mil

$$18$$

Chapter 18: Post-Traumatic Growth

You didn't choose trauma. You didn't ask for PTSD. But here you are, carrying wounds that may never fully heal.

The question isn't whether trauma changed you—it did. The question is: who are you becoming because of it?

This final chapter is about post-traumatic growth: the possibility that you can emerge from trauma not just surviving, but transformed in meaningful ways. Not "back to normal," but forward to something new.

Post-traumatic growth doesn't erase the pain. It doesn't make the trauma "worth it." But it offers a way to integrate your experiences, find meaning, and build a life where trauma is part of your story—but not the whole story.

What is Post-Traumatic Growth?

Post-traumatic growth (PTG) is the positive psychological change that can occur as a result of struggling with highly challenging life circumstances.

It's not about bouncing back (resilience). It's about bouncing forward—becoming a different, and in some ways stronger, person because of what you've endured.

Research shows PTG can occur in five domains:

1. Greater appreciation for life

You don't take things for granted anymore. Small moments matter.

You're grateful for ordinary days.

2. Deeper relationships

Your relationships become more authentic. You value the people who stuck by you. You let go of superficial connections.

3. Increased personal strength

You know you can survive the worst. You're stronger than you thought.

"If I survived that, I can survive this."

4. New possibilities

Trauma closed some doors, but it opened others. You explore new interests, careers, identities.

5. Spiritual or philosophical growth

You've wrestled with life's biggest questions: Why do bad things happen? What's the meaning of suffering? What matters most? You've developed a deeper worldview.

Post-Traumatic Growth Is Not:

- A silver lining ("Everything happens for a reason")
- Toxic positivity ("Just focus on the positive!")
- A requirement ("If you don't grow from trauma, you failed")
- The opposite of PTSD (you can experience both simultaneously)

You can grow from trauma and still struggle. Both can be true.

The Path to Post-Traumatic Growth

Growth doesn't happen automatically. It requires intentional work.

Step 1: Process the Trauma

You can't grow from trauma you're avoiding. Growth begins after you've done the hard work of processing what happened through therapy (CPT, PE, EMDR).

You have to face it, feel it, and integrate it before you can move forward.

Step 2: Make Meaning

Meaning-making is central to PTG. It's not about justifying the trauma

("It happened for a reason"), but about finding purpose despite it.

Questions to explore:

- What did this experience teach me about myself?
- What values matter most to me now?
- How have my priorities shifted?
- What do I want my life to stand for moving forward?

Some people find meaning through:

- **Service**: Using their experience to help others
- **Advocacy**: Fighting to prevent others from experiencing similar trauma or to improve systems
- **Creativity**: Expressing their journey through art, writing, music
- **Relationships**: Investing deeply in the people who matter
- **Spirituality**: Connecting with something larger than themselves

Step 3: Challenge Your Assumptions

Trauma shatters your core beliefs about the world:

- "The world is safe." (It's not.)
- "Good things happen to good people." (They don't.)
- "I'm in control." (You're not.)

PTG involves rebuilding a worldview that accommodates these harsh truths without becoming cynical or hopeless.

New, more nuanced beliefs might be:

- "The world has danger, but also beauty and connection."
- "Life is random and unfair, but I can still choose how I respond."
- "I can't control everything, but I can control my actions and
- values."

This rebuilding takes time. Be patient with yourself.

Step 4: Connect with Others

Growth is rarely a solo journey. Connection with others—especially those who understand your trauma—facilitates PTG.

- Support groups let you see others' growth, which shows you it's possible
- Mentorship (being mentored and mentoring others) creates purpose and meaning
- Authentic relationships remind you that you're valued beyond your trauma

Step 5: Take Action Aligned with Your Values

Growth requires living differently, not just thinking differently.

If you value service, volunteer.

If you value family, invest time in relationships.

If you value honesty, stop hiding your struggles.

If you value courage, do something that scares you.

Action creates identity. You become who you practice being.

Domains of Post-Traumatic Growth

Let's explore each domain in detail.

1. Greater Appreciation for Life

Before trauma, you may have moved through life on autopilot. After trauma, you can't. You're acutely aware that life is fragile, temporary, precious.

Examples:

- A sunrise isn't just pretty—it's a gift
- A conversation with your child isn't routine—it's sacred
- An ordinary Tuesday is a victory

This appreciation can coexist with grief. You can be grateful to be alive while also mourning what you've lost. Both can be true.

Practice: Daily gratitude

Each night, write three things you're grateful for today. They don't have to be big. "I had hot coffee. My dog greeted me at the door. I didn't have nightmares last night."

Gratitude doesn't erase pain, but it creates balance.

2. Deeper, More Authentic Relationships

Trauma reveals who your people are. Some disappear. Others show up in ways you didn't expect.

After trauma, superficial relationships feel empty. You crave depth, authenticity, realness.

You're also better at boundaries. You know your limits. You don't waste energy on people who drain you.

Examples:

- You're honest about your struggles instead of pretending everything's fine
- You ask for help when you need it
- You tell people you love them instead of assuming they know

- You let go of toxic relationships without guilt

Practice: Deepen one relationship

Choose one person you value. Have a real conversation. Be vulnerable.

Share something true. Ask about their inner life, not just surface stuff.

3. Increased Sense of Personal Strength

"If I survived that, I can survive this."

Trauma proves you're tougher than you thought. You've endured what you once believed would destroy you. You're still here.

This doesn't mean you're invincible. It means you have evidence that you can face hard things and survive.

Examples:

- Starting a new job feels less scary because you've survived worse
- A breakup hurts, but you know you've survived loss before
- Public speaking is nerve-wracking, but you've faced actual danger

Practice: Reflect on your resilience

Write: "I survived ______. That proves I am ______."

Example: "I survived three combat deployments and years of PTSD. That proves I am resilient, capable of enduring immense pain, and worthy of recovery."

4. Exploration of New Possibilities

Trauma closes some doors. You might not be able to return to your old job, your old identity, your old life.

But it also opens doors you didn't know existed.

Examples:

- A medically retired soldier becomes a therapist specializing in
- veteran PTSD

- A firefighter who can't fight fires anymore becomes a peer support
- specialist
- A veteran starts a nonprofit helping other veterans transition

Trauma often clarifies what matters. You stop wasting time on things that don't align with your values.

Practice: Explore something new

Try something you wouldn't have tried before trauma. A new hobby, a class, a volunteer opportunity. Give yourself permission to reinvent.

5. Spiritual or Philosophical Growth

Trauma forces you to confront life's biggest questions:

- Why do bad things happen?
- What is the meaning of suffering?
- Is there a God? If so, why did this happen?
- What matters most?

Some people lose their faith. Some deepen it. Some find new spiritual or philosophical frameworks.

PTG isn't about having answers. It's about wrestling with the questions and developing a worldview that gives your life meaning.

Examples:

- A veteran who lost faith in organized religion develops a personal
- spiritual practice
- An atheist finds meaning in secular humanism and service to others
- A believer's faith becomes more nuanced and less dogmatic

Practice: Reflect on your worldview

Write: "Before trauma, I believed _____. Now, I believe _____."

Example: "Before trauma, I believed the world was fair and God protected good people. Now, I believe the world is random and chaotic, but I can still choose to act with compassion and integrity."

Stories of Post-Traumatic Growth

From Despair to Advocacy

Sergeant Maria Lopez developed severe PTSD after military sexual trauma.

For years, she struggled in silence, ashamed and isolated. After intensive therapy, she began speaking publicly about MST, advocating for better reporting systems and survivor support. She testified before Congress. She started a nonprofit connecting MST survivors with resources.

"I will always carry the trauma," Maria says. "But I've used it to create change. I've helped other survivors feel less alone. That gives my pain purpose."

From Firefighter to Peer Mentor

John Davis was a firefighter for 15 years before PTSD from repeated traumatic calls forced him to medically retire. He spiraled into depression and substance use. After treatment, he became a certified peer support specialist, working with other first responders struggling with PTSD.

"I lost my career, but I found a new mission," John reflects. "I help people survive the same hell I went through. That matters more than I ever imagined."

From Combat Veteran to Artist

After three deployments, Corporal David Chen couldn't articulate his experiences in words. He started painting—dark, abstract pieces exploring trauma, loss, and resilience. His art was exhibited at veteran centers and galleries. Through art, he processed his trauma and connected with other veterans who saw themselves in his work.

"I thought I lost everything in war," David says. "But I found a way to express what I couldn't say. Art saved my life."

PTG and Ongoing Struggle

Post-traumatic growth doesn't mean you're "cured." You can grow from trauma and still have bad days, bad weeks, bad months.

You can be grateful for your life and also wish the trauma never happened.

You can be stronger because of what you endured and still hate that you had to endure it.

Growth and struggle coexist. That's not hypocrisy. That's the complexity of being human.

Living Forward

The rest of your life starts now.

You can't change what happened. You can't undo the trauma. But you can choose what happens next.

You can:

- Build relationships rooted in authenticity
- Pursue work that aligns with your values
- Help others navigate their own struggles
- Live with intention and gratitude
- Create meaning from your pain

This doesn't make the trauma "worth it." Nothing makes it worth it.

But it means the trauma doesn't get the final word. You do.

Your story isn't over. This is just the end of this chapter.

What you write next is up to you.

Practical Exercises

Exercise 1: PTG Reflection

For each domain, write one way you've grown (or could grow):

1. Greater appreciation for life:

Example: "I no longer take my morning coffee for granted. I savor it."

2. Deeper relationships:

Example: "I tell my kids I love them every day now. I used to assume they knew."

3. Increased personal strength:

Example: "I survived PTSD. I know I can handle difficult conversations now."

4. New possibilities:

Example: "I started volunteering with a veteran mentorship program."

5. Spiritual/philosophical growth:

Example: "I've developed a daily meditation practice that grounds me."

Exercise 2: Meaning Statement

Write a one-paragraph statement about the meaning you've created from your trauma.

Example:

"My PTSD from combat forced me to confront my own mortality and the randomness of life. It shattered my illusions of control and safety. But through that shattering, I've learned what truly matters: my family, my integrity, and using my experience to help other veterans. I will always carry the wounds of war. But I also carry wisdom, resilience, and a commitment to living purposefully. My trauma doesn't define me, but it has shaped who I'm becoming."

Exercise 3: Future Self Letter

Write a letter to yourself five years from now.

Describe:

- Where you hope to be in your recovery
- What kind of person you want to become
- What you want to have accomplished
- What you hope to have let go of
- Seal it. Open it in five years.

Exercise 4: Growth Action Plan

Choose one action aligned with each domain of PTG. Commit to doing it this month.

Example:

1. Appreciation: Start a daily gratitude journal

2. Relationships: Have a vulnerable conversation with my spouse

3. Personal strength: Sign up for that class I've been afraid to try

4. New possibilities: Research volunteer opportunities

5. Spiritual growth: Attend one religious/spiritual service or read one philosophy book

Final Thoughts

PTSD is a wound, not an identity. You are not your trauma. You are not your diagnosis. You are not broken beyond repair.

You are a person who experienced something terrible and is finding a way forward. That takes courage. That takes strength. That takes showing up day after day, even when it's hard.

The road ahead won't be easy. There will be setbacks. There will be days you want to give up. But you've survived the worst. You can survive this. And maybe—just maybe—you'll discover that you're not just surviving.

You're growing. You're becoming. You're moving forward.

Your unseen march isn't over. But you're not marching alone anymore.

Keep going.

Wayne's Insight

"When I started this journey, I was broken. I genuinely believed PTSD had destroyed me and that the best I could hope for was to survive. I couldn't imagine growth. I couldn't imagine joy. I couldn't imagine purpose beyond just getting through each day.

"But here I am, years later, and I'm not the same person I was before my deployments. I'm not the same person I was in the worst of my PTSD.

I'm someone new—someone shaped by trauma but not defined by it.

"I appreciate life differently now. I don't waste time on things that don't matter. I tell my family I love them every single day. I hug my kids longer. I watch sunsets and actually see them.

"I've found a new mission: helping other veterans navigate PTSD. I mentor younger vets. I speak openly about my struggles. I'm not ashamed anymore. My trauma gave me the ability to connect with people in their darkest moments and tell them: 'I've been there. I survived. You can too.'

"Do I still have hard days? Absolutely. Do I still have nightmares sometimes? Yes. Do I still carry guilt and grief? Always. But I also carry strength, wisdom, and purpose I didn't have before. "I'll never say my trauma was 'worth it.' That's not how it works.

But I will say this: I'm proud of who I'm becoming despite it. I'm proud of the life I'm building. I'm proud of the husband, father, veteran, and mentor I am today.

"If you're reading this and you're still in the thick of it, I need you to know: growth is possible. You won't be who you were before. But that's okay. You get to decide who you become next.

"Your story isn't over. This is just the beginning of what's possible.

"Keep marching forward. I'm marching with you."

Chapter 18 End Notes
& References

Tedeschi, R. G., & Calhoun, L. G. (1996). "The Post-traumatic Growth

Inventory: Measuring the Positive Legacy of Trauma." Journal of Traumatic Stress, 9(3), 455-471.

Tedeschi, R. G., & Calhoun, L. G. (2004). "Post-traumatic Growth: Conceptual Foundations and Empirical Evidence." Psychological Inquiry, 15(1), 1-18.

Pietrzak, R. H., Goldstein, M. B., Malley, J. C., Rivers, A. J., Johnson, D. C., & Southwick, S. M. (2010). "Post-traumatic Growth in Veterans of Operations Enduring Freedom and Iraqi Freedom." Journal of Affective Disorders, 126(1-2), 230-235.

Shakespeare-Finch, J., & Lurie-Beck, J. (2014). "A Meta-Analytic Clarification of the Relationship Between Post-traumatic Growth and Symptoms of Post-traumatic Distress Disorder." Journal of Anxiety

Disorders, 28(2), 223-229.

Calhoun, L. G., & Tedeschi, R. G. (2006). *Handbook of Post-traumatic

Growth: Research and Practice.* Lawrence Erlbaum Associates.

Park, C. L. (2010). "Making Sense of the Meaning Literature: An Integrative Review of Meaning Making and Its Effects on Adjustment to Stressful Life Events." Psychological Bulletin, 136(2), 257-301.

Joseph, S., & Linley, P. A. (2005). "Positive Adjustment to Threatening

Events: An Organismic Valuing Theory of Growth Through Adversity."

Review of General Psychology, 9(3), 262-280.

Tedeschi, R. G., Shakespeare-Finch, J., Taku, K., & Calhoun, L. G.

(2018). *Post-traumatic Growth: Theory, Research, and Applications.*
Routledge.

Epilogue: The Unseen March Continues

Let's recap the core messages of this book, because they're worth repeating.

PTSD is real. It's not a weakness. It's not your fault. It's a medical condition with biological, psychological, and social dimensions. Your brain and body respond to trauma in predictable ways. You're not broken. You're injured. And injuries can heal.

PTSD is treatable. Evidence-based treatments work. CPT, PE, EMDR, medication when needed, these aren't just buzzwords. They're proven interventions that help 60-80% of people who try them. Recovery is possible. Not guaranteed. Not easy. But it is possible.

You are not alone. Thousands of military and first responders live with PTSD. Millions of people worldwide. The shame and isolation you feel? Everyone feels that. The belief that no one understands? Wrong. We understand. We've been there. You're not alone.

Help-seeking is strength, not weakness. The hardest thing you'll ever do is walk into that first therapy appointment and admit you need help. That takes more courage than anything you did in uniform. Don't let anyone, including yourself, tell you otherwise.

Recovery isn't linear. Bad days will come even after good weeks. Setbacks happen. That's not failure. That's recovery. Keep going.

Your life can be more than survival. You can build a life worth living. Not perfect. Not painless. But meaningful, connected, purposeful. You deserve that life. And you can have it.

These aren't platitudes. These are facts, backed by research and thousands of recovery stories.

The question is: what will you do with these facts?

The march didn't end when you left the military or retired from first responder work. It didn't end when you got diagnosed with PTSD. It doesn't end when you finish this book.

The march continues.

Every day you get out of bed despite the nightmares—that's the march.

Every time you go to therapy even though it's painful—that's the march.

Every moment you choose connection over isolation—that's the march.

Every time you help another veteran or first responder find their way—that's the march.

You're not marching in formation anymore. You're not marching to someone else's orders. You're marching to the rhythm of your own healing, at your own pace, toward a destination you get to choose.

And you're not marching alone. Thousands of us are out here, carrying our own wounds, finding our own way forward. We're your tribe. We're your people. We've got your six.

The march is long. The terrain is hard. But you're tougher than you know.

Keep marching.

Follow @breakingranksblog on social media platforms

┌─────┐
│ **19** │
└─────┘

APPENDIX A

Community Resource Directory

All resources are free or low-cost. No referral required. For immediate crisis support, call or text 988.

COMMUNITY RESOURCE DIRECTORY

PEER SUPPORT

- **VA PTSD Support Groups**
  Free, clinician-led • va.gov
- **Vet Center Groups**
  No enrollment required • vetcenter.va.gov
- **Wounded Warrior Project**
  Peer support + wellness • woundedwarriorproject.org
- **Team RWB**
  Fitness + social connection • teamrwb.org

VETERAN SERVICE ORGS (VSOs)

- **Disabled American Veterans**
  Claims help, transport • dav.org
- **Veterans of Foreign Wars**
  Benefits, grants, community • vfw.org
- **American Legion**
  Advocacy + programs • legion.org
- **Iraq & Afghanistan Vets (IAVA)**
  Advocacy + mental health • iava.org
- **Team Rubicon**
  Mission-driven service • teamrubiconusa.org
- **The Mission Continues**
  Volunteer + leadership • missioncontinues.org

FIRST RESPONDER ORGS

- **Code Green Campaign**
  EMS mental health resources • codegreencampaign.org
- **Firefighter Behavioral Health**
  Peer support + prevention • ffbha.org
- **Badge of Life**
  Law enforcement support • badgeoflife.com
- **NAMI**
  Support groups + resources • nami.org

EMPLOYMENT & EDUCATION

- **Hire Heroes USA**
  Free job search + resume help • hireheroesusa.org
- **American Corporate Partners**
  Corporate mentorship • acp-usa.org
- **VA Vocational Rehab (VR&E)**
  Training + employment • va.gov
- **GI Bill**
  Education benefits • va.gov/education

FAMILY SUPPORT

- **PTSD Family Coach App**
  Free VA app for families • mobile.va.gov
- **Give an Hour**
  Free counseling for families • giveanhour.org
- **Blue Star Families**
  Community + programs • bluestarfam.org
- **Natl Military Family Assoc.**
  Resources + support • militaryfamily.org

SPECIALIZED SUPPORT

- **VA MST Coordinators**
  At every VA facility
- **Safe Helpline (DoD)**
  MST support • 1-877-995-5247
- **Women Veterans Call Center**
  1-855-829-6636
- **VA LGBTQ+ Coordinators**
  At every VA facility
- **OutServe-SLDN**
  Legal support • outserve-sldn.org

VA APPS (FREE)

Figure 17.2 — Community Resource Directory. All organizations listed are free or low-cost. No referral is required to call any of these numbers.

APPENDIX B

Personal Crisis Safety Plan

A crisis safety plan is one of the most powerful tools you can have. Complete this now—before you need it. Keep it somewhere accessible: on your phone, posted at home, or given to a trusted person. The warning signs and coping steps are yours alone; the crisis lines at the bottom are universal.

MY PERSONAL CRISIS SAFETY PLAN

Fill this in. Keep it somewhere you can find it fast.

⚠ MY WARNING SIGNS

When I notice these signs, I need to use my plan:

1.
2.
3. _______________________________

▮ MY COPING STEPS (DO THESE FIRST)

Before calling anyone, try these on my own:

1.
2.
3. Box breathing: Inhale 4 · Hold 4 · Exhale 4 · Hold 4

▮ MY PERSONAL SUPPORT CONTACTS

People I can call when I need to talk:

Name: ______________ Phone: ______________
Name: ______________ Phone: ______________
Name: ______________ Phone: ______________

▮ CRISIS LINES (USE IF ABOVE DON'T HELP)

Immediate professional support — 24 hours a day:
988 Suicide & Crisis Lifeline → Call or text 988
Veterans Crisis Line → Call 988, press 1 / Text 838255
Safe Call Now (First Responders) → 1-206-459-3020

My name: ______________ Date completed: ______________

Share this plan with someone you trust.

Appendix B — Personal Crisis Safety Plan. Fill in your warning signs, coping steps, and personal contacts. The crisis lines at the bottom are pre-filled and active 24 hours a day.

APPENDIX C

Grounding Techniques Quick Reference

When a trigger hits, the thinking brain goes offline. This card gives you four techniques you can use without having to remember instructions. Practice each one before you need it—so that when the moment comes, your body already knows what to do.

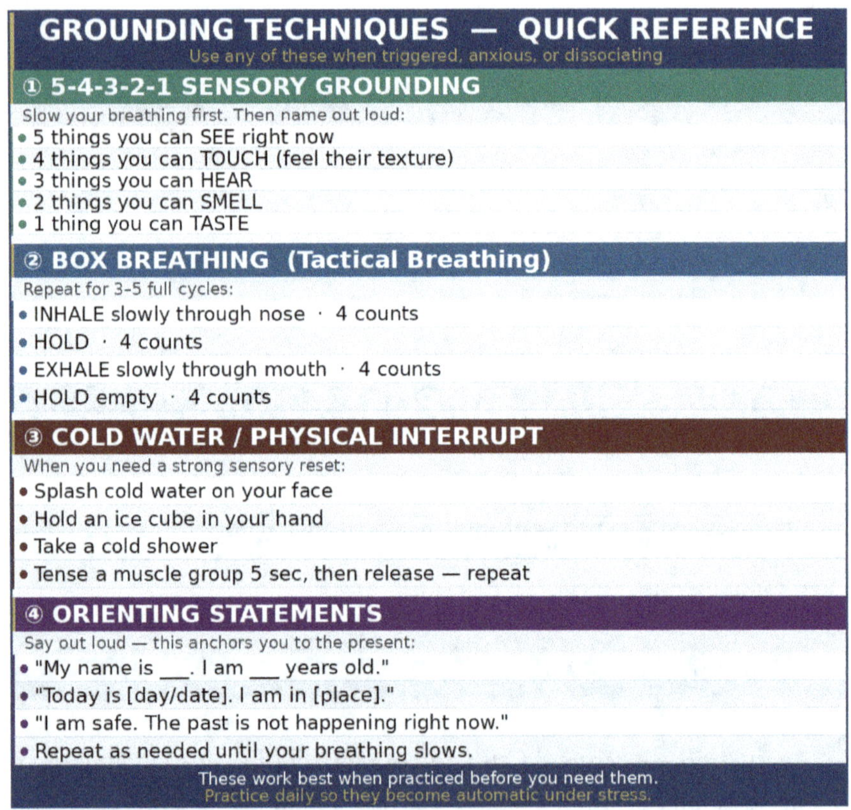

Appendix C — Grounding Techniques Quick Reference. All four techniques from Chapter 4. Keep this accessible during high-stress periods. The goal is to practice daily until these responses become automatic.

APPENDIX D

My Support Network Map

Recovery is not a solo mission. Research consistently shows that the strength and diversity of your support network is one of the strongest predictors of PTSD recovery outcomes. Use this map to identify who is in each ring of your network—and where the gaps are. See Chapter 17 for organizations that can fill any ring that is currently empty.

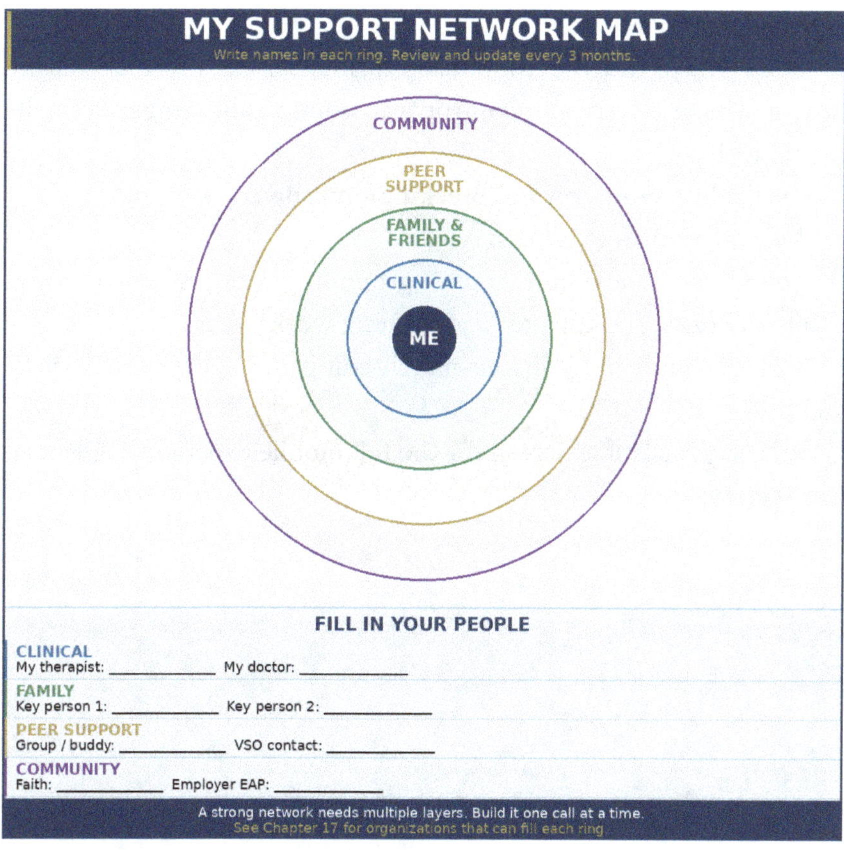

Appendix D — My Support Network Map. The closer the ring to the center, the more immediate the relationship. A resilient network has people in

every ring. Fill in names and update every three months as your network grows.

MORE BOOKS FROM THE AUTHOR

UNTIL THE WELL RUNS DRY

Non-Fiction

A comprehensive guide to mental health in the African American community, addressing stigma, cultural barriers, and pathways to healing.

SWEETWATER RECKONING

Fiction - Thriller

Book One of the Marcus Johnson thriller series. A former Marine turned private investigator confronts corruption and danger in small-town Florida.

Available on Amazon and BreakingRanksBooks.com

Mental Wellness Health App

Your Free Companion App — grounding tools, mood tracking, crisis resources, and Chapter 5 journaling worksheets.

Visit big-sarge.blog/unseen-march-companion · Password: [rucksack]

Add to your Home Screen for the full mobile experience. QR scan code below:

UNSEEN
MARCH

www.ingramcontent.com/pod-product-compliance
Lightning Source LLC
Chambersburg PA
CBHW070855160726
48004CB00003B/1087